What Is the *Depression* Workbook?

Depression affects many people. Its symptoms can be mild, moderate, or severe. It might last for a short while or for longer periods of time. This workbook will help you learn about and address symptoms of *mild to moderate* depression. It is designed to be flexible: you can either complete exercises in sequence or focus on those that meet your needs.

"There is hope, even when your brain tells you there isn't."

—John Green

SECTION 1

What Is Depression?

Many of us experience depression at some point in life. Recognizing the signs and sources of it can help us learn to manage it.

EXERCISE 1

Depression: More Than Sadness

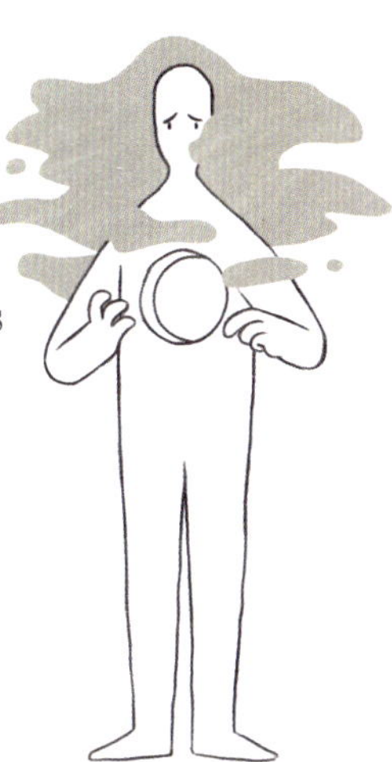

We all feel "down" at times, but while sadness subsides, depression tends to linger. Depression can disrupt our sleep and eating habits and can make concentrating difficult. Depression also includes feelings of emptiness, apathy, low self-esteem, and hopelessness. It may include a lack of interest in activities, physical slowness or restlessness, strong feelings of shame, and at its darkest, thoughts of death or a desire to die. Important differences between sadness and depression have to do with the strength of these feelings and how long they last.

Read the following scenarios and mark them with an "S" or a "D" if they represent sadness or depression. The first is done for you.

Scenario	
Tyrone was laid off. He fought tears while packing his desk, but he resolved to start looking for a new job the next day.	S
For many weeks after her grandmother's funeral, Toni had little interest in seeing her friends. Within a few months, she started accepting invitations and resumed most of her activities.	
DeShawn was laid off from his job. After months of sending out résumés and not getting interviews, he stopped looking for work and started drinking heavily.	
Leah applied to one college, her "dream school," and didn't get in. She started sleeping later and later every morning and was not motivated to make alternative plans.	
Rick's girlfriend broke up with him. He spent several days in bed, ignoring calls and texts. Within a few months, his friends persuaded him to go out and start dating again, which he did.	

How are sadness and depression similar and different for you?
Explain your experience.

When we feel trapped in a lingering state of apathy or emptiness, we may be experiencing depression.

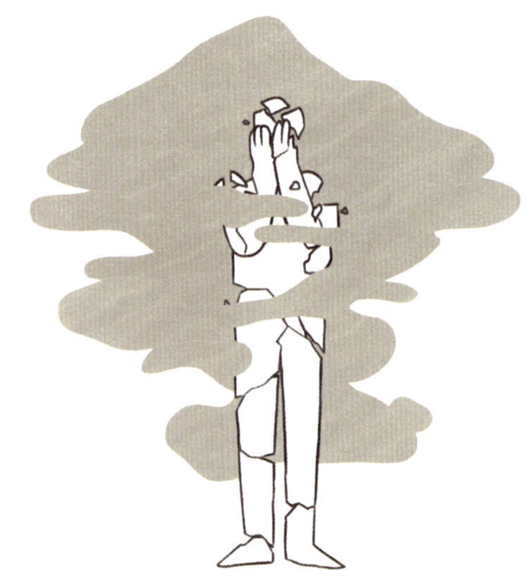

"It's so difficult to describe depression to someone who's never been there, because it's not sadness. I know sadness. Sadness is to cry and to feel. But it's that cold absence of feeling—that really hollowed-out feeling."

—J. K. Rowling

EXERCISE 2

Symptoms of Depression

We all experience depression differently, but there are common symptoms that many people have. We can experience them off and on throughout life or all the time. Sometimes these symptoms are very strong, and sometimes they are mild.

Here are some symptoms that are common when we feel depressed. Check the ones you notice in yourself. If you notice symptoms that aren't listed, write them in the "other" spaces.

- ☐ I feel a deep sadness.
- ☐ I'm not motivated to start or finish anything.
- ☐ I don't enjoy activities like I used to.
- ☐ I blame myself when things go wrong.
- ☐ I feel pessimistic about the future.
- ☐ I don't like myself.
- ☐ I have no energy.
- ☐ I feel guilty or ashamed most of the time.
- ☐ I often think about death.
- ☐ I drink or use other substances more than normal.
- ☐ Other:
- ☐ I feel like I'm being punished.
- ☐ I have trouble concentrating.
- ☐ I get into fights with other people.
- ☐ I seem to move more slowly than I used to.
- ☐ I have problems sleeping—I wake up throughout the night, can't sleep well, or sleep too much.
- ☐ I have problems with food—I either overeat or don't eat enough.
- ☐ I have lost interest in sex/intimacy.
- ☐ I'm more irritable than normal.
- ☐ I feel worthless.
- ☐ I don't see any point in doing things.
- ☐ Other:

Of the symptoms you marked, which bother you the most?

What do you think would change if you didn't have the symptoms you marked?

The first step is recognizing the signs that we are struggling with depression. Once we realize what the problem is, we can take steps to start feeling better.

I'm irritable.
I can't sleep.
I drink more.

It Takes Practice

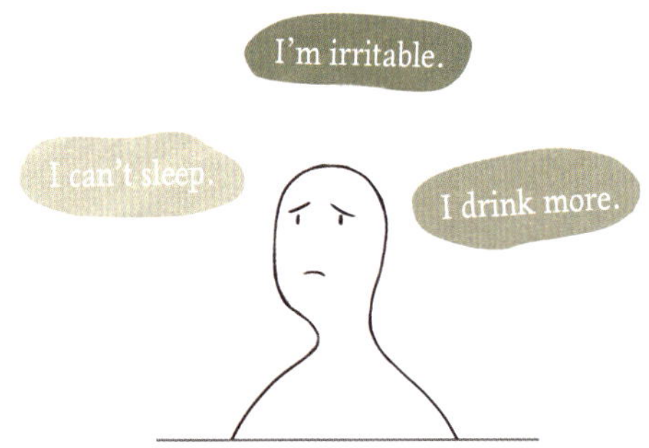

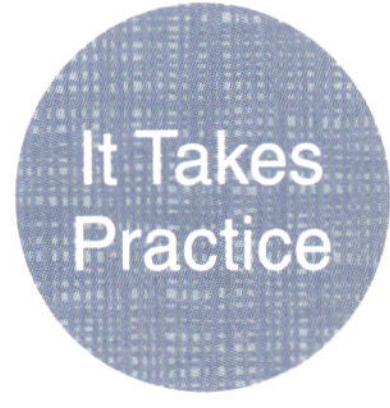

Keep a journal, noting how you feel each day. Rate your depression symptoms on a scale of mild, moderate, or strong.

EXERCISE 3

What Is Depression Like for Me?

Depression affects us mentally, physically, emotionally, and spiritually. We each experience it in different ways that are unique to us.

Mental Experiences of Depression

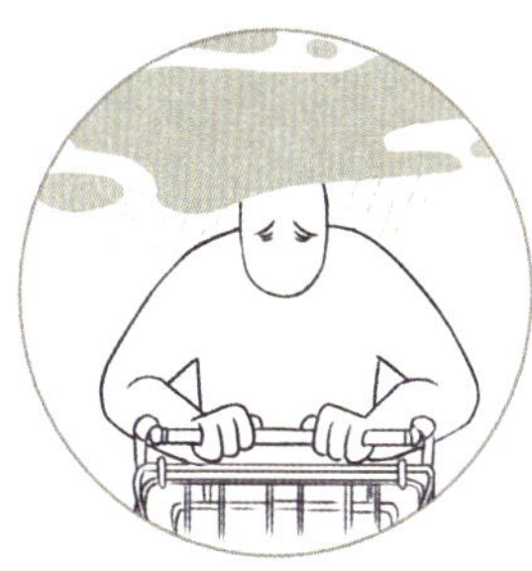

Sometimes, depression can bring about negative thoughts about ourselves or the world. We might have a dark outlook on life or sense that things are going wrong and will continue to do so. We might revisit difficult memories over and over again or even put ourselves down with negative "self-talk."

In the bubbles below, write some words or phrases that show the difference between your thoughts when you're not depressed and your thoughts when you are.

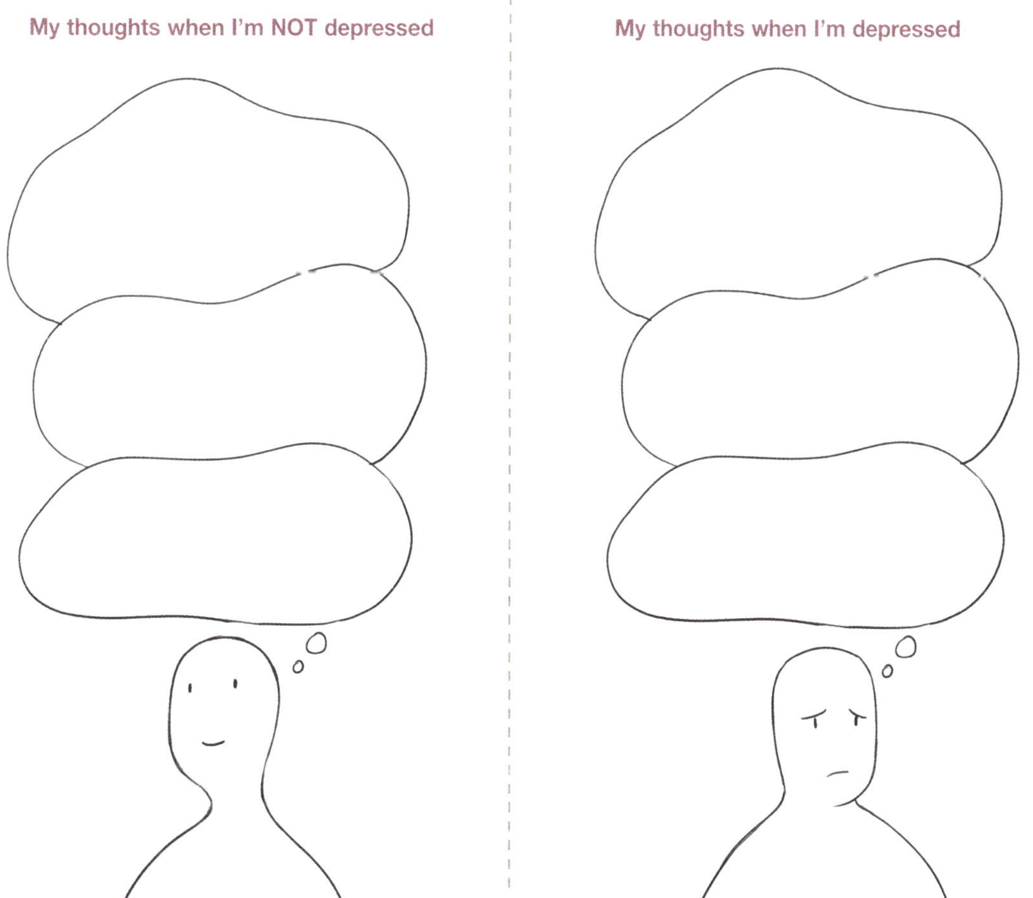

Complete the following sentence with words that describe your thoughts in depression.

My thoughts when I'm depressed seem to center on ______________________________

____

____

Physical Experiences of Depression

Depression can sap our energy, making us feel like doing nothing at all. It can make us feel drained, heavy, or weighed down. It can also feel like a sadness that doesn't cease—we may feel like we're trapped or folding in on ourselves.

Shade in the batteries to compare your typical energy level to that in depression.

My typical energy level

My energy level in depression

Complete the following sentences with words that describe how you feel physically when depressed.

When I'm depressed, my energy level is ______________________________

Physically, depression makes me feel ______________________________

____

____

Emotional Experiences of Depression

While sadness is a common feeling associated with depression, several other emotions are linked to it as well. We may feel a range of emotions at different levels of intensity when we're depressed.

Circle the emotions that you typically feel when you're depressed. If there are feelings you notice that aren't listed here, write them in the clouds below.

upset	hopeless	despondent	angry
irritable	numb	frustrated	furious
wistful	lonely	helpless	confused
morose	guilty	ashamed	gloomy
fearful	indifferent	frantic	anxious

What emotions associated with depression would you most like to change?

Spiritual Experiences of Depression

For many of us, depression brings on feelings of doubt and makes us question our purpose in life.

Circle the sentences below that apply to you when you feel depressed.

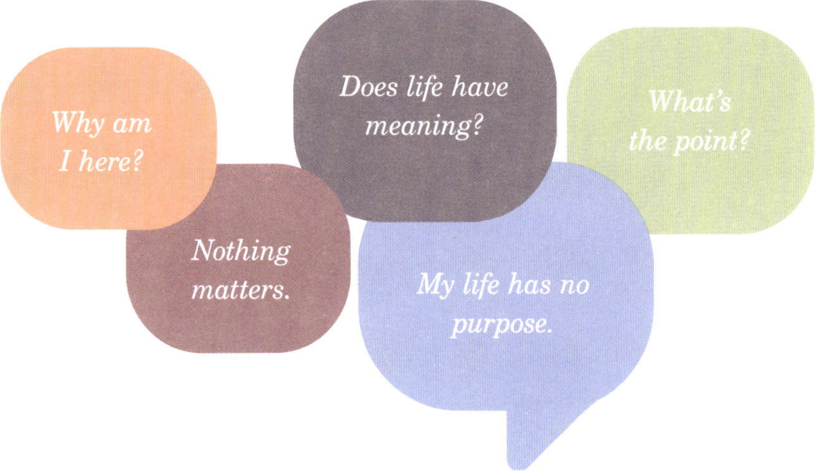

What differences do you notice when you're *not* depressed compared to when you are? Consider your thoughts, emotions, physical feelings, and spirituality.

It is important to realize that these experiences with depression are not something we just need to "get used to." Depression is treatable. There are things we can do to make ourselves feel better—mentally, physically, emotionally, and spiritually.

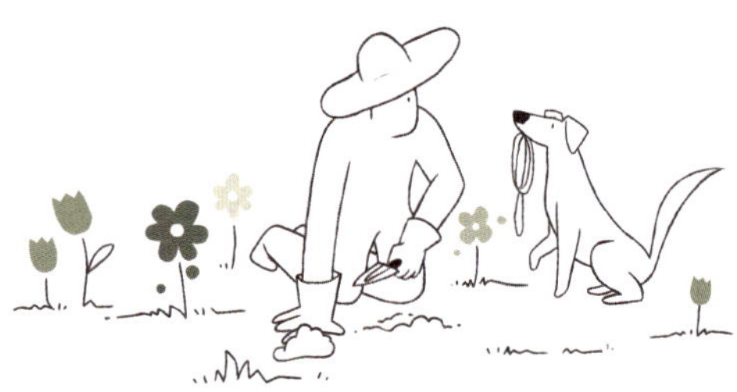

"No storm, not even the one in your life, can last forever. The storm is just passing over."

—Iyanla Vanzant

EXERCISE 4

Sources of Depression

Depression may come from multiple factors in a person's life. Some of us may be susceptible to feeling depressed because of our genes and biological background. If a close biological relative has had depression, we are more likely to become depressed ourselves.

In the circles below, note any biological relatives that you're aware of who have experienced depression. Then answer the questions on the next page.

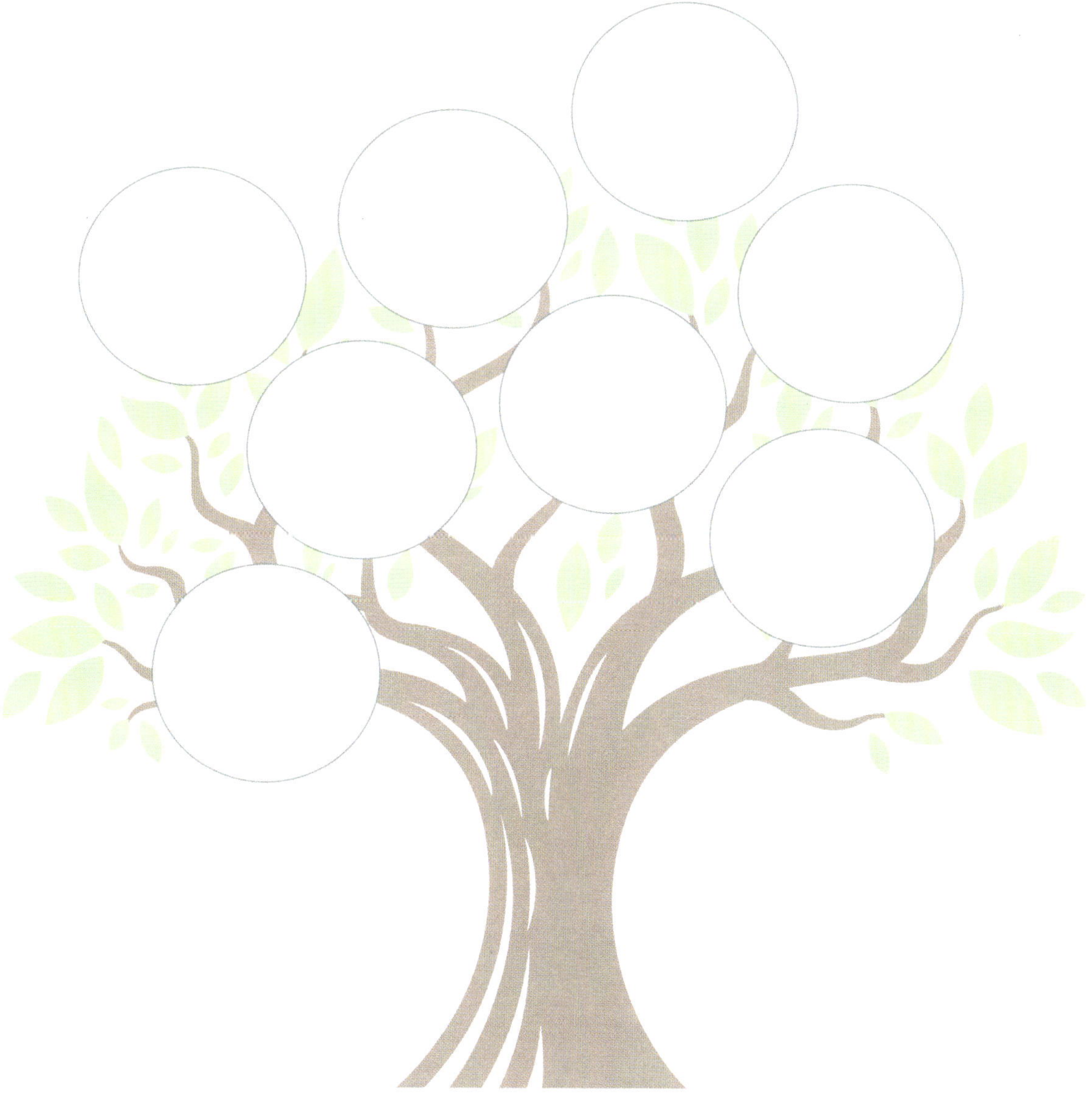

How did depression affect them mentally, physically, emotionally, or spiritually?

What impact, if any, do you think their depression has had on you and your emotional health today?

Some of us may struggle with depressed feelings because of our personal history and life experiences, including difficulties such as divorce or past abuse.

What are some challenging events you have experienced in life, and how do they affect your feelings of depression today?

In addition to our background and early life experiences, stress in life can also cause depression. Sometimes we become depressed because of circumstances that feel too challenging to work through. Sometimes we become depressed because we feel trapped with no good decisions to make.

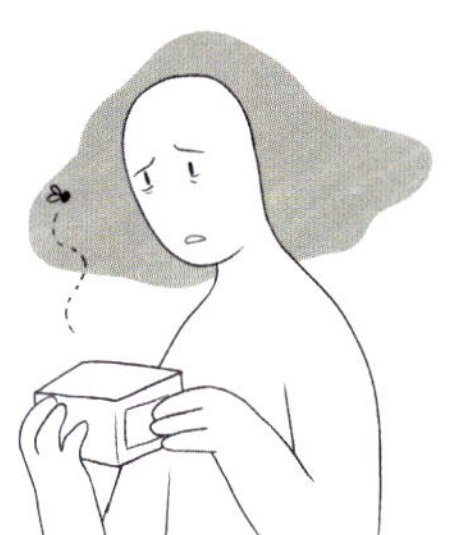

Check the areas of your life that are stressful for you and explain how they contribute to your depression.

- [ ] **Finances**

____

____

____

- [ ] **Romantic relationship/partner**

____

____

____

- [ ] **Social life**

____

____

____

- [ ] **Work or school**

____

____

____

- ☐ **Living arrangement**

- ☐ **Obligations outside of work/school**

- ☐ **Substance use/addiction**

- ☐ **Family or children**

By understanding what influences our feelings of depression, we can start to address them, find ways to overcome them, and ultimately reduce our symptoms and improve our mood.

SECTION 2

Depression in My Life

Depression affects our thoughts, feelings, and actions. Reflecting on the ways it influences our thinking patterns and behavior is the first step in learning to manage it.

EXERCISE 5

Coping and Choices

Depression isn't comfortable. It can even be painful. Sometimes, we make choices or do things to stop feeling pain or discomfort when we're depressed. We try to avoid these feelings, push them away, or shut them down.

Have you noticed yourself doing any of the following things to try to "escape" feelings of depression? Circle those that apply to you. In the blank spaces, add any other things you do.

sleeping much later than usual, or taking long naps	drinking more than usual	smoking/vaping more often than usual	using substances like marijuana or painkillers
having risky sex	buying unnecessary things	spending excessive time on the internet or watching television	pretending to be happy on the "outside"
eating more or eating less	picking or cutting skin	isolating yourself from other people	not returning phone calls, emails, or texts
acting aggressive, or trying to control other people	overworking, or immersing yourself in tasks without taking breaks		

These methods of dealing with the pain of depression have two important things in common:

1. ***They're temporary.*** Any relief they offer is short-lived, and they don't make problems go away.
2. ***They're harmful.*** In one way or another, each of these behaviors ultimately makes life harder for us—whether by introducing or worsening an addictive habit, affecting our health, or allowing us to deny a problem.

While these coping strategies may feel helpful in the moment, they don't help us face our underlying problems. In fact, they can even make things *worse.* They can send us down paths that reinforce depression, making it even harder to overcome.

Describe some other unhelpful coping strategies you have used to try to manage your depression in the past.

____

____

____

What happened when you used these coping strategies? How have they affected your life?

____

____

____

Reflecting on unhelpful ways we have coped with depression might seem like it could give us more negative thoughts—but really, it helps us get clear about what *doesn't* work. Once we have this insight, we can become more open to taking steps that *will* work.

"Numbing the pain for a while will make it worse when you finally feel it."

—J. K. Rowling

EXERCISE 6

The Impact of Depression

Sometimes, if we're dealing with depression, we may feel like we are the only ones affected by it. After all, we have the troubling thoughts and the deep sense of unhappiness. But our depression plays out in our relationships with others, whether we realize it or not.

In the diagram below, shade the areas of your life that you think have been affected by your depression. Think about choices you have made, how you've interacted with other people, or feedback you've received.

school
friendships
work, job
relationships with parents, guardians
relationships with extended family
relationships with children
relationships with siblings
relationships with coworkers
faith, spiritual community
money, finances
sports, hobbies, activities, community
relationship with significant other, spouse

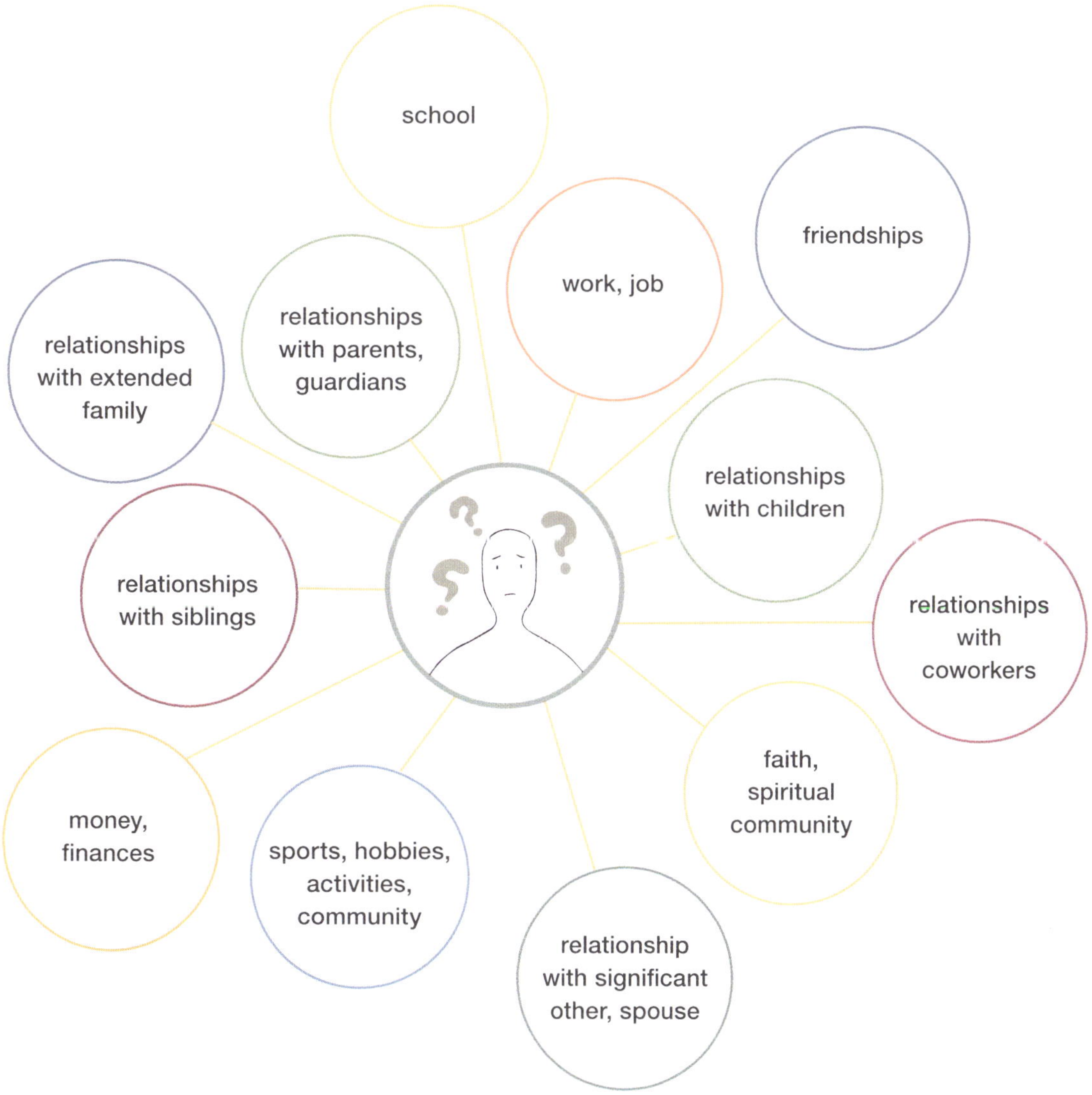

In the following table, list the top three people or areas of your life that have been affected by your depression. Write how they have been affected and what might change if you felt better. Feel free to add areas that aren't represented in the diagram on page 15.

Who or what is affected?	How?	What might change if you felt better?

The reality is, our depression affects how we respond to the world and relate to others. Looking at these impacts doesn't mean we should feel worse about our depression. It just means there are lots of reasons to try to start feeling better—not just for ourselves, but for others too.

"No matter how bad things are right now. No matter how stuck you feel. No matter how many days you've spent crying and wishing things were different. No matter how hopeless and depressed you feel. I promise you that you won't feel this way forever. Keep going."

—Helen Wilson

EXERCISE 7

Negative Self-Talk

When we're depressed, we often find ourselves thinking negatively about ourselves and our lives. These negative thoughts often get repeated over and over in our minds. This is called "negative self-talk."

Here are some examples.

> Chris dropped out of school when they were sixteen. Now twenty-eight, Chris has trouble finding a job they enjoy. "I'm just not smart," they say to themself.

> Addie has raised three kids and has a busy advertising career. But she finds herself fixating on an insulting comment a friend made at a reunion long ago. "I'm a loser," she thinks.

When we repeat negative thoughts to ourselves, we may start to believe them. Eventually, these repeated thoughts become automatic—we stop thinking about what it is we're saying to ourselves because we've turned these thoughts into beliefs about who we are.

Think about the way you talk to yourself and answer the following questions.

How would you describe most of the themes you have about yourself? (Check one.)

very negative | mostly negative | neutral | mostly positive | very positive

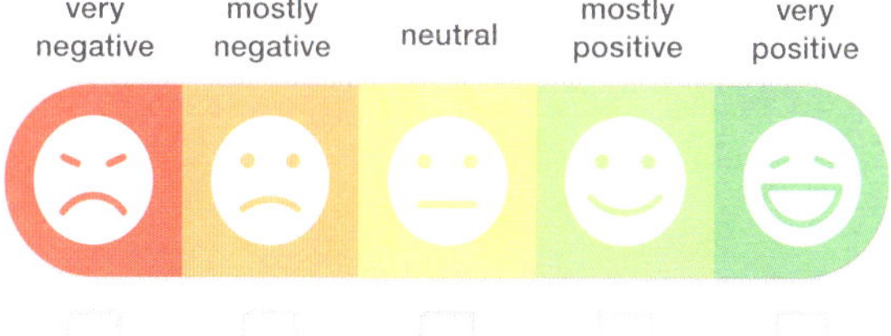

☐ ☐ ☐ ☐ ☐

What are some of the common themes in your negative self-talk?

____

____

____

What would you most like to change about your negative self-talk?

All of us struggle with negative self-talk. When we feel depressed, that negative self-talk can be even louder. But just as we can change the station on a radio, we can change the self-talk we listen to. In the boxes below, write some new things you could say to yourself in the following areas.

Who you are

Your life circumstances

Mistakes you've made in the past

Your future

Your relationship with others

It Takes Practice

Whenever you experience negative self-talk during your day, pause and replace that negative thought with a positive one. The more you practice this, the easier it will become.

EXERCISE 8

Linking Thoughts and Feelings

We tend to overlook the connection between our thoughts and feelings. We often think our feelings "just happen"—that they seem to come up instantly, and we don't always know why. When we're depressed, it's useful to look at the link between our thoughts and feelings because it's possible to use our thoughts to change our feelings.

Events don't *cause* feelings. Our feelings are caused by thoughts we have *about* events. And it's those resulting feelings that drive our behaviors.

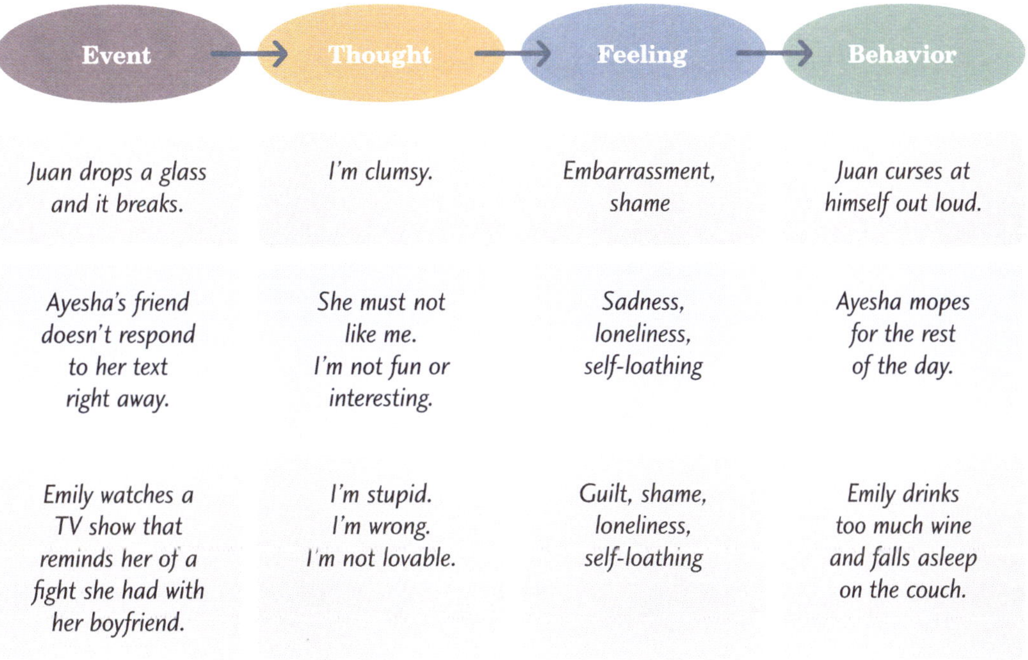

At no time do our feelings bypass our thoughts! A person may think, "My boyfriend broke up with me, so I got depressed." But there was a *thought* or *thoughts* that led to feeling depressed. The thoughts might be

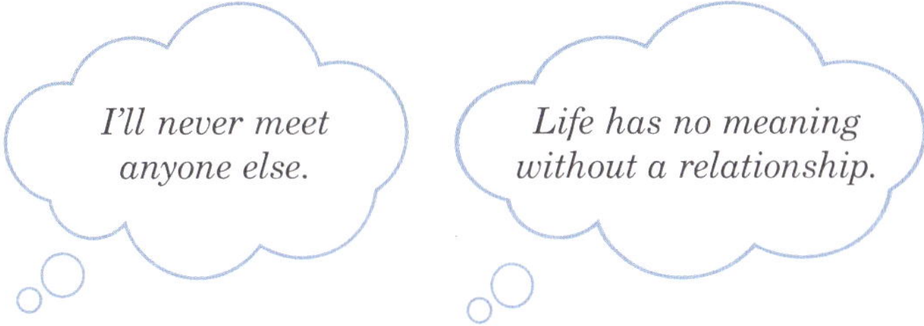

How would this person's depressed feelings change if they had these more positive thoughts, as shown in the thought bubbles?

This experience is hard. I need to take care of myself.

I'm sorry he broke up with me, but maybe it's for the best.

And how would this person's behavior change?

They might exercise more and spend more time with friends. They might be sad for a while, but then start dating again.

Let's practice this skill of identifying the thoughts behind our feelings.

Think about a recent event in which you found yourself feeling depressed. In the chart below, fill in the event and the thought, feeling, and behavior that occurred. *Tip:* It is often easier to start with behavior or feeling and work backward to identify the thought you had about the event. Then answer the questions on the next page.

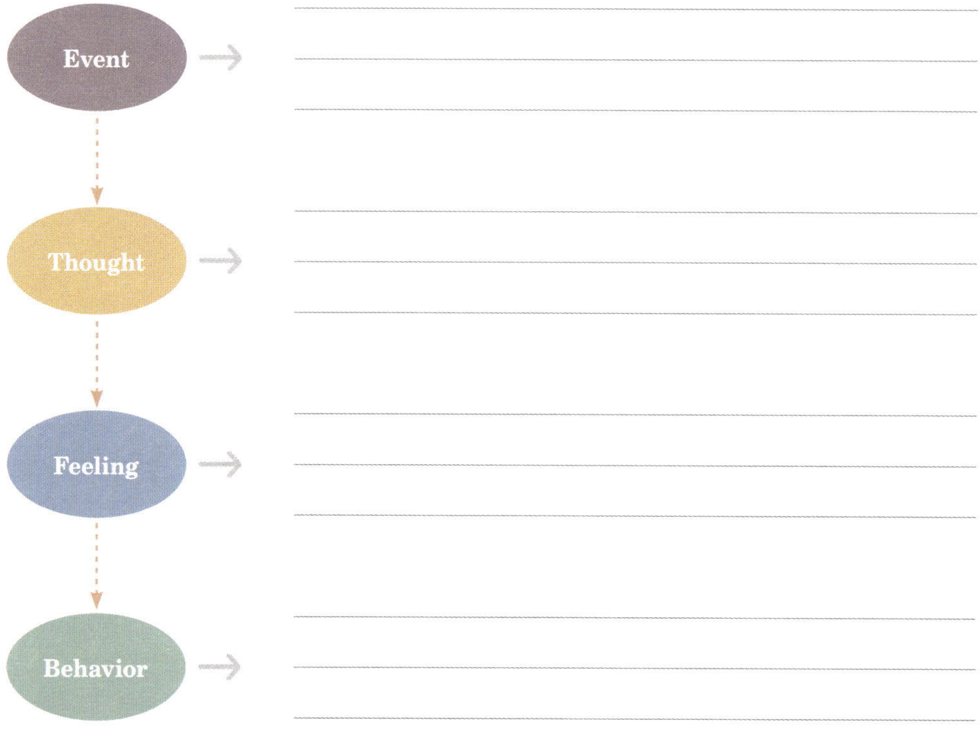

How do you think your depression would be affected if you focused on changing your thoughts?

What are some common thoughts you would change?

Understanding how our thoughts affect our feelings, and in turn affect our behavior, gives us a powerful strategy to overcome depression. We can see that changing our thoughts can profoundly change our feelings and behaviors.

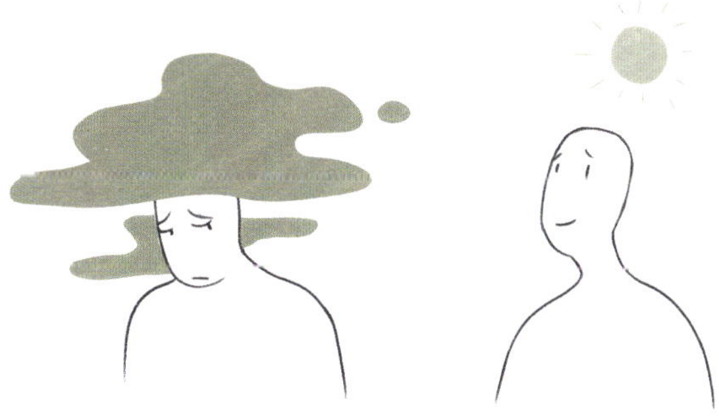

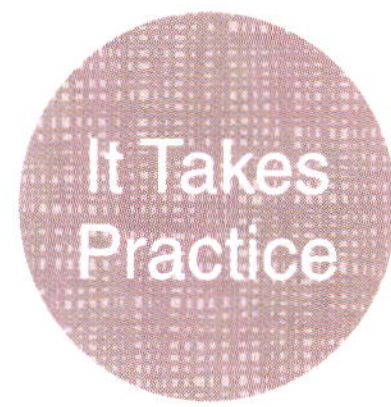

Keep a Thought Journal for a week. Write down any negative thoughts you are having whenever you are feeling depressed. Don't judge the thoughts, just note them in your journal.

EXERCISE 9

Core Beliefs: The Thoughts behind Our Thinking

Core beliefs are what we believe to be true about ourselves, other people, and the world. We all have core beliefs about how things work and how things *should* work, and we have judgments about many things—including ourselves.

The world is out to get me.
I'm lovable.
People are generally nice.

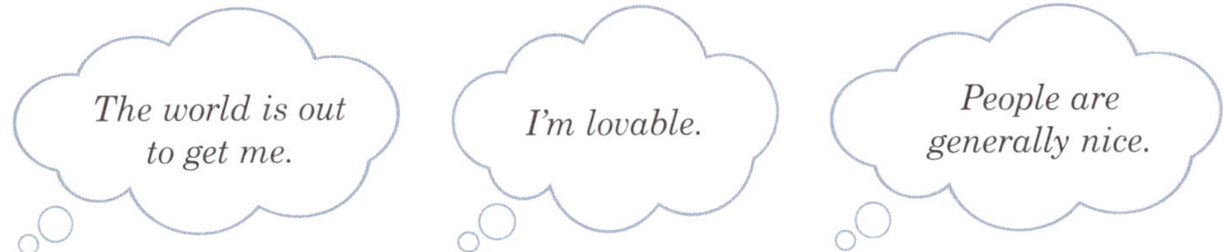

Core beliefs are the thoughts *behind* our thoughts. They might be beliefs we learned as children or beliefs we developed over time.

Event
Core Belief
Thought
Feeling
Behavior

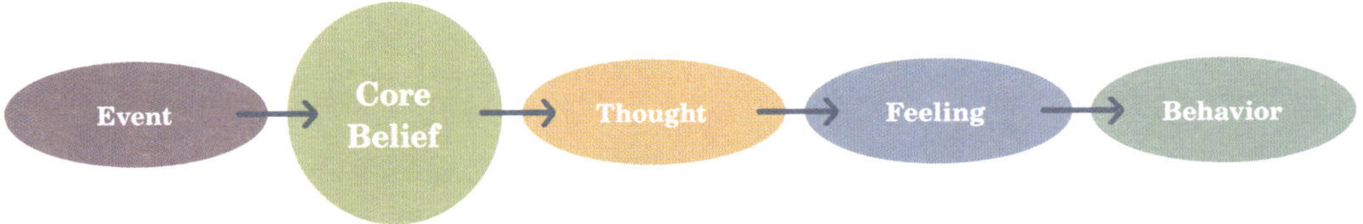

We don't think about our core beliefs; they're automatic. They affect how we think, feel, and behave even when we don't realize it.

Start to explore your core beliefs by writing words and phrases that come to mind to complete the following sentences. Some examples are given.

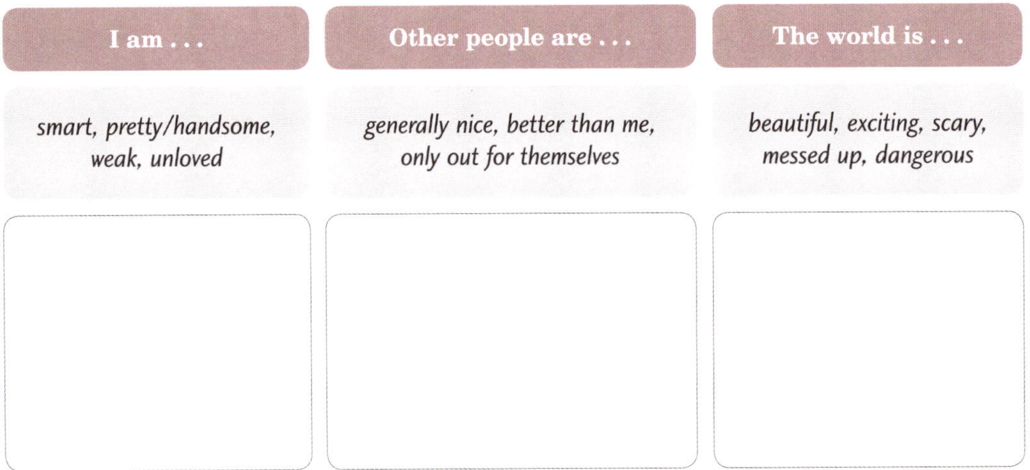

I am . . .	Other people are . . .	The world is . . .
smart, pretty/handsome, weak, unloved	*generally nice, better than me, only out for themselves*	*beautiful, exciting, scary, messed up, dangerous*

When we dig deeper, we may find we have some surprising core beliefs that have a profound effect on our feelings of depression. They can also have a profound effect on our life overall.

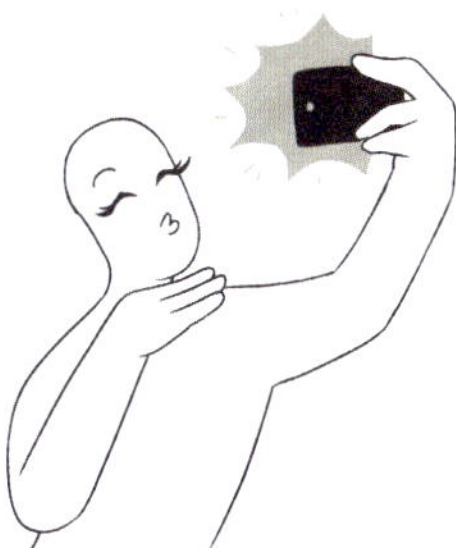

Reflect on a negative core belief you have about yourself. Start by writing this core belief in the box below. Then answer the questions that follow.

My core belief

1. How might this core belief affect you at work or school?

2. How might this core belief affect the way you assert yourself with others?

3. How might this core belief affect you in social situations?

4. How might this core belief affect you in romantic relationships?

5. How might this core belief affect your view of your future?

Negative core beliefs can keep our depression going, like fuel in the tank of a car. But we can learn to challenge and replace our negative core beliefs. Let's practice now.

On the lines below, write three negative core beliefs that affect your feelings of depression. Then write a positive core belief that could replace it. An example is done for you.

> **Negative core belief:** *I can't trust anyone.*
>
> **New positive core belief:** *There are trustworthy people in the world. I just need to look for them.*

Negative core belief: ______________________________

____

New positive core belief: ______________________________

____

• • •

Negative core belief: ______________________________

____

New positive core belief: ______________________________

____

• • •

Negative core belief: ______________________________

____

New positive core belief: ______________________________

____

Challenging and replacing our negative core beliefs takes practice and focused effort, but it can be done. If we work at changing our core beliefs, changed thoughts, feelings, and behaviors will follow.

EXERCISE 10

Selective Focus

We tend to see the world with a narrow viewpoint when we're depressed—like looking through the wrong end of a telescope. We focus on negative memories and ideas about ourselves, our life, and others.

When we consider only the negative, eventually we come to *expect* and *believe* we'll find only negative things. It's like we intentionally choose what we're looking for.

Read the following scenario:

> Jamal and Jane are coworkers. On the way to lunch, they pass their supervisor, who is reading from a folder of papers and doesn't look up as she passes by.

Jane thinks, "She looks busy."

Jamal thinks, "She didn't look up or say hi. Why didn't she say anything? What did I do?"

Which person may have a negative viewpoint? ______________________

Which person is looking at things in a more positive way? ______________________

When we view situations positively, it's called "looking at the world through rose-colored glasses." What color are our glasses when we're depressed?

What would it take to shift the color of the glasses you wear? What would change if you chose to focus on the positive?

____

____

____

____

____

In and around the lenses of this pair of glasses, write some positive words and phrases about yourself and your life. If you have trouble coming up with ideas, ask someone you trust to help.

When we're feeling depressed, it may take extra effort to see the positive—but it's there! The more we focus on the positive, the better we'll feel.

It Takes Practice

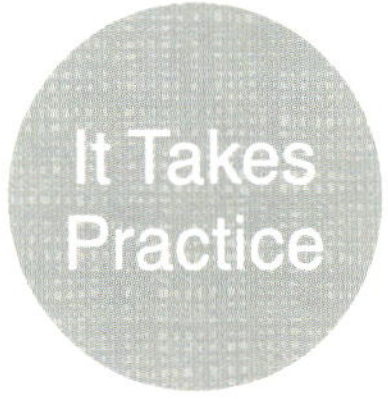

Every morning and evening, think of three positive things in your life. Write them down.

EXERCISE 11

Distorted Thinking

Sometimes we use shortcuts in our thinking that aren't helpful. Called "thinking distortions," these patterns negatively affect the way we look at things. Not only can these distortions mislead us, they can also deepen our depression.

Here are ten thinking distortions that people with depression commonly use.

Thinking Distortion	What It Means	Examples
Jumping to Conclusions	**Mind reading:** You assume others think negatively about you. **Fortune telling:** You predict things will turn out badly without looking at the evidence or likelihood.	**Mind reading:** *He looked down when I spoke. He must not like me.* *She didn't come to lunch. She must be mad at me.* **Fortune telling:** *I know she won't listen to me.* *I know he won't care about me.*
"Should" Statements	You criticize yourself or others with phrases like "should have," "ought to," and "must."	*I should never have said that.* *I ought to do this better.*
Magnification or Minimization	You blow little things way out of proportion and/or you downplay important, meaningful events.	**Magnification:** *I'm running late, so I may as well stay home. I'm going to get fired anyway.* *My problems are worse than everyone else's.* **Minimization:** *I only slept four hours this afternoon.* *My depression isn't that bad!*

table continued on next page

Thinking Distortion	What It Means	Examples
Emotional Reasoning	You have a feeling and then look for a way to justify it.	*I feel stupid, so I must be stupid.* *I feel depressed, because my life has no meaning.*
Extreme or "All or Nothing" Thinking	You view matters in absolute, black-and-white ways.	*Everybody always . . .* *I will always be depressed.*
Over-generalization or "Always or Never" Thinking	You view a single negative event as a never-ending pattern of defeat and pessimism.	*I failed my test. I can never do anything right.* *My marriage ended. I'll never find love again.*
Personalization and Blame	You blame yourself for something you were not responsible for, or you blame others without noting your part in the problem.	*It's my fault my husband has a problem with alcohol.* *If you had kids like mine, you'd be depressed too!*
Labeling	Instead of focusing on the problem, you label and judge yourself to be the problem.	*I'm late for work—I'm a terrible worker!*
Selective Focus	You focus on the negatives and dismiss the positives.	*But that's just one good thing—and there are so many bad things.*
Mental Filter	Good things or good qualities "don't really count," or you dismiss the source.	*She's just saying that to be polite.* *He's only telling me he likes me because he wants something.*

Most of us use these thinking distortions from time to time, but when we're depressed, we use them more frequently.

Which thinking distortions do you use most often? Write them below.

Thinking distortion 1: ______________________________

Thinking distortion 2: ______________________________

Thinking distortion 3: ______________________________

Describe a recent event where you used one of these thinking distortions. The event could be something you said or did, or something someone else said or did to you.

____

____

____

____

Which thinking distortion did you use? ______________________________

Now, consider the same event and describe how you might have looked at it differently—in a way that doesn't distort what happened.

____

____

____

____

When we change our distorted thinking, much like changing the lenses in our glasses, we get a clearer, more honest, and more useful view of our life and ourselves.

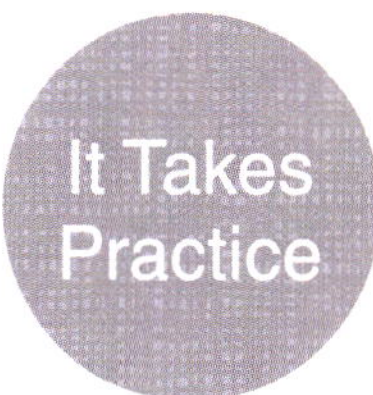

Keep a Thought Journal for several days. Note when you have a distorted thought and identify which thinking distortion it is. Try to come up with a more positive thought to put in its place.

Facing Depression

SECTION

3

From challenging or detaching from our negative thoughts to adopting healthy habits like exercising and getting enough sleep, there are many things we can do to manage our depression and release its hold over our lives.

EXERCISE 12

Replacing Negative Thoughts with Positive Ones

It's often our thoughts that lead to feelings of depression. If we want to change our feelings, we need to replace our negative thoughts with more positive ones. Here's an example:

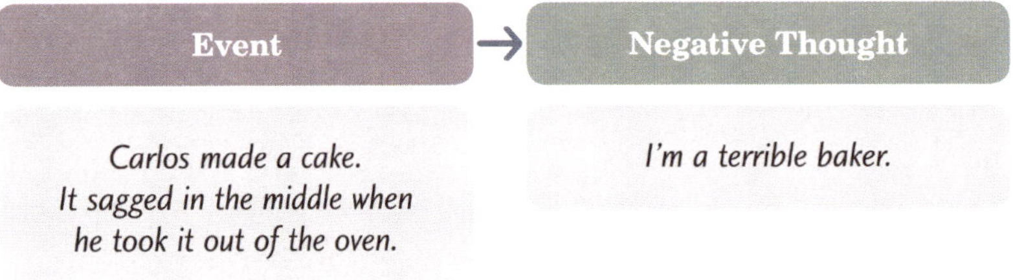

Answer the following questions.

How did Carlos most likely *feel* after he *thought* he was a terrible baker?

Imagine that Carlos replaced his negative thought with this alternative positive thought:

> *I was talking on the phone and baking at the same time. I'm a better baker when I'm not distracted.*

How would Carlos most likely feel after thinking this more positive thought?

Alternative positive thoughts can change our feelings. Here's an example.

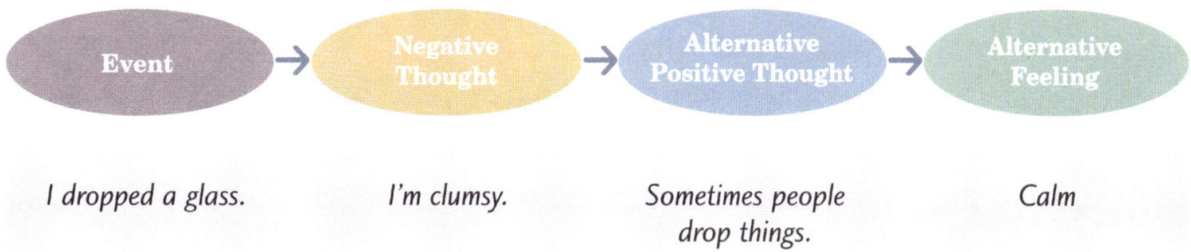

List a recent event that resulted in you having some negative, depressing thoughts. List the negative thoughts. Then list one or more alternative positive thoughts you could have had. What are some different feelings you might have had because of the more positive thought? Write these alternative feelings in the spaces that follow.

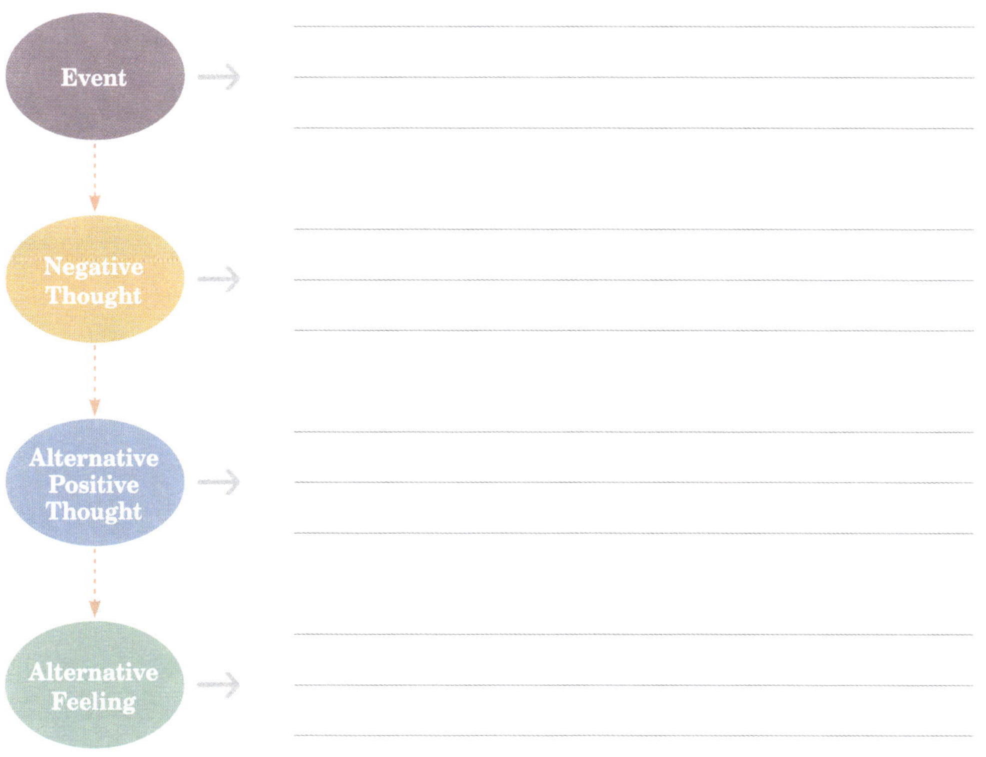

Let's practice this some more. Write three negative thoughts you've had recently. Then challenge each negative thought with two related positive thoughts.

Negative thought: ______________________________

Positive thought 1: ______________________________

Positive thought 2: ______________________________

Negative thought: ______________________________

Positive thought 1: ______________________________

Positive thought 2: ______________________________

Negative thought: ______________________________

Positive thought 1: ______________________________

Positive thought 2: ______________________________

The great news is we have power over our thoughts. We can choose which thoughts we think. As we go about our day, we can practice replacing our negative thoughts with positive ones.

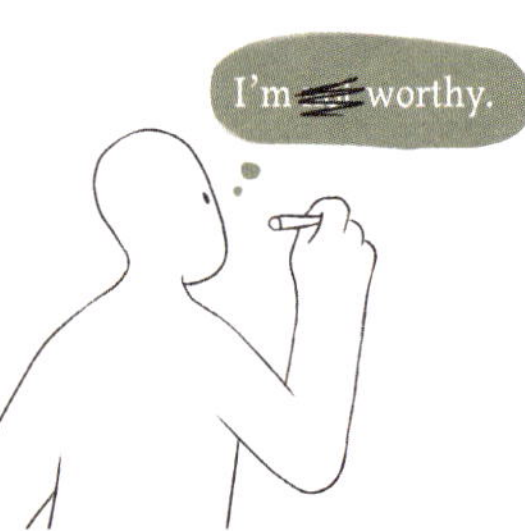

"If you don't like something, change it; if you can't change it, change the way you think about it."

—Mary Engelbreit

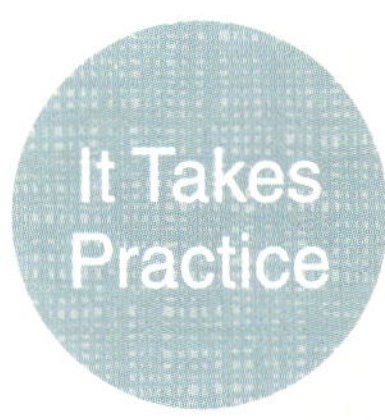

When you catch yourself having a negative thought, challenge yourself to replace it with a positive one instead.

EXERCISE 13

Detaching from Negative Thoughts

When we feel caught up in our negative thoughts, it can be helpful to detach from them. Instead of challenging them or trying to come up with alternative thoughts, just let them go.

How does this work?

Imagine your negative thoughts written out on cards.

Imagine yourself shuffling through the cards. You examine them, turn them over . . .

Then you crumple them up one by one and toss them in the trash.

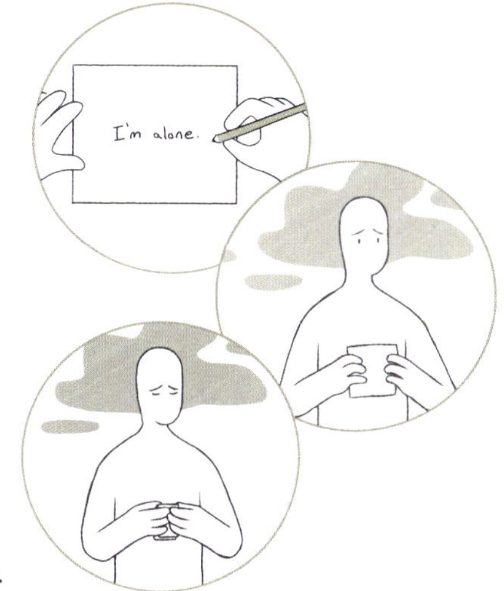

This is what we mean by detachment:
Observing a thought and then calmly letting it go.

Think of some of the negative thoughts you've had lately that you would like to "let go." Write them in the spaces below.

Thought 1	Thought 2	Thought 3

You could rewrite each of these negative thoughts on a piece of paper, then crumple them up and throw them away.

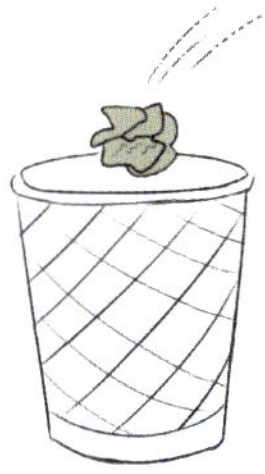

Detaching can be a little easier if we learn to pull the energy and power out of our negative thoughts.

One way to do this is to precede a thought with these words: "I'm having the thought that . . ." For example, "*I'm having the thought that* I should always appear calm and confident."

Experiment with other "front-end" phrases you can use to observe your thoughts and take away some of their emotional energy.

In the following table, the left column has some possible phrases. Fill in the second column with a negative thought you're having that you want to detach from. An example is provided.

Phrase	Negative Thought
Now my mind is having the thought that . . .	*I should have said something different.*
The thought that just popped into my mind is . . .	
I notice that once again I'm thinking . . .	
I'm having the thought that . . .	

Notice the effect of using these phrases. Adding the extra words puts a little space between us and our thoughts. In a subtle way, these statements remind us that we are more than our thoughts. Thoughts come and go a million times a day. But the essential *you*—your capacity to simply be aware of thoughts—always remains.

Not all thoughts are created equal. Some thoughts serve us well. We want to keep those. But other thoughts are unhelpful. We can detach from them and let them go.

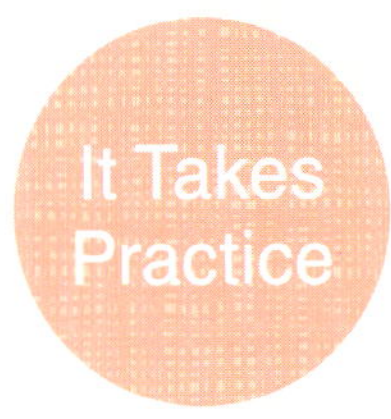

Practice using these phrases as much as possible for a day. Then expand to two days and so on. Eventually they will become second nature.

EXERCISE 14

Using Our Wise Mind

When our feelings are overwhelming, it can seem like they "take over," and there's nothing we can do to stop them. But it's our thoughts that cause our feelings—and we can do something about our thoughts. Even when things seem really bad, we can think about how to respond. We can accept difficult events without being overcome by negative emotions.

Sometimes we think rationally, with logic. Other times, we're more emotional. It's important that we use both our "rational mind" and our "emotional mind" to effectively respond to situations we face. If we use only our emotional mind, we may not reason well, and we risk overreacting to situations. If we use only our rational mind, we may neglect our intuition.

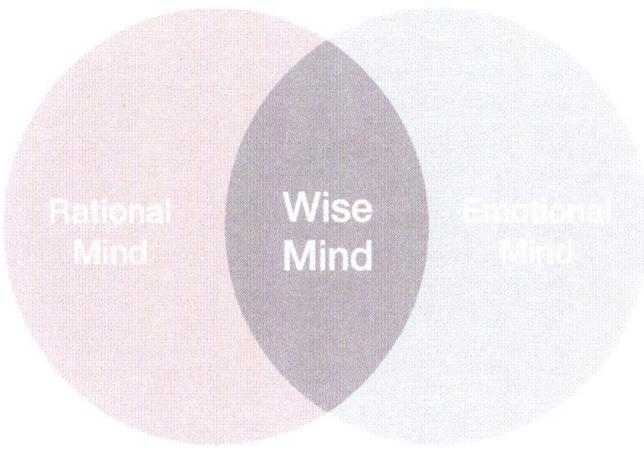

When we pause, observe, and think about something rationally *and* emotionally, we are using our **"wise mind."** You can think about it in the following way:

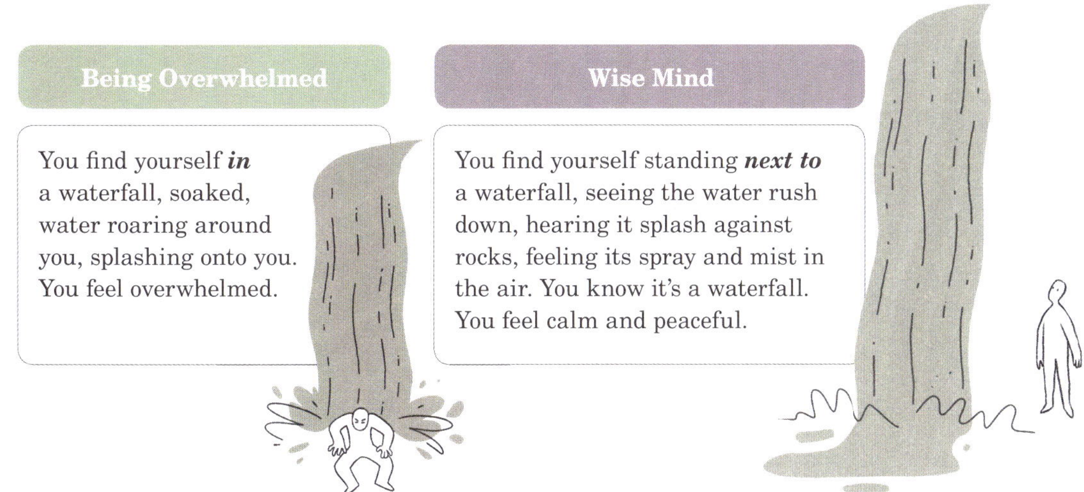

Look at the following examples. What would be a wise mind response if these people could stand *outside* the waterfall of emotion? An example is provided.

Being Overwhelmed	Wise Mind
After a stressful day at work, Katie stopped at the grocery store and bought three cartons of ice cream to eat instead of dinner.	*Katie had a stressful day at work. She was tempted to buy several cartons of ice cream at the store that evening. After pausing, she decided to eat dinner and have only one serving of dessert.*
Carson was excited after a job interview, but was told the job was given to someone else. He got depressed and started smoking weed.	
Shante's doctor told her she has a serious medical issue. She felt overwhelmed and cried uncontrollably all evening.	

Answer the following questions.

How are your overwhelming feelings of depression affecting your actions at this time?

How could you change your actions if you paused and considered a wise mind approach?

The scenarios below offer a way to look at this wise mind process of finding perspective and thinking before we respond:

Scenario 1: **Event • Response**

Scenario 2: **Event ——— Response**

Both the • and the ——— **signify time**. The dot is an ***instant response***. The dash represents a ***pause to observe***, think of alternative thoughts, and decide what to do.

One simple way to extend the time between an event and our response is by using our breath. Breathe in and count to three, and breathe out and count to four. Keep repeating as needed.

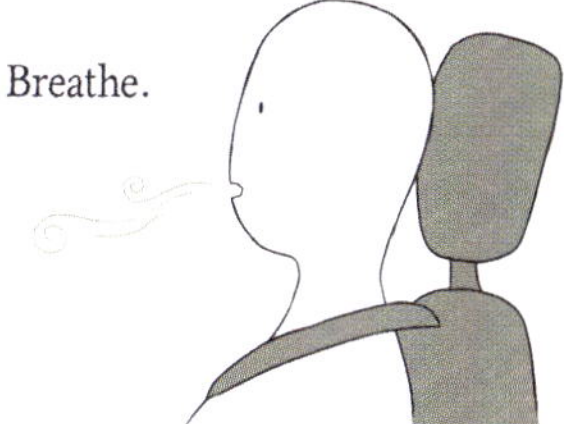

There are many good breathing techniques, but you may find that this one is simple enough to remember and powerful enough to give you time to use your wise mind.

When we're used to living "under the waterfall" of our depressing emotions, it can be comforting to see a better way to live that gives us more control.

"Between stimulus and response there is a space. In that space is our power to choose our response. In our response lies our growth and our freedom."

—Viktor Frankl

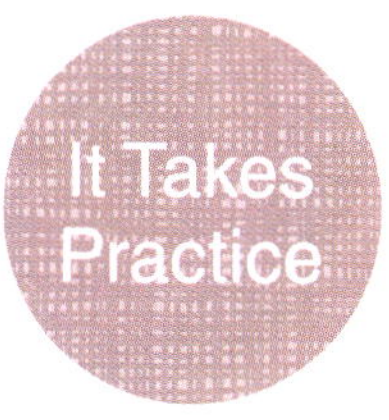

When something happens where you typically respond with depressed thoughts, take a deep breath and go into wise mind. Pause and think about how to respond.

EXERCISE 15

Healthy Activities for Depression

When we're depressed, our energy level often goes down and we do less. Or, following the "path of least resistance," we start doing things that are not helpful to us.

Mark the things you do when you're depressed.

- ☐ I sleep a lot.
- ☐ I eat more than usual.
- ☐ I eat less than usual.
- ☐ I don't call or text people.
- ☐ I procrastinate.
- ☐ I don't exercise.
- ☐ I smoke/vape more than usual.
- ☐ I shop more than usual.
- ☐ I drink more than usual.
- ☐ I don't enjoy my usual activities.
- ☐ I watch more TV than usual.
- ☐ Other: ______________________

____

____

For many of us, doing these things can prolong or worsen our depression because they allow us more time to focus on our negative thoughts, or they make us feel worse because they aren't healthy or productive.

It can be helpful—even life-changing—to raise our level of activity and challenge our sluggish behaviors with coping strategies that are energizing and mentally engaging.

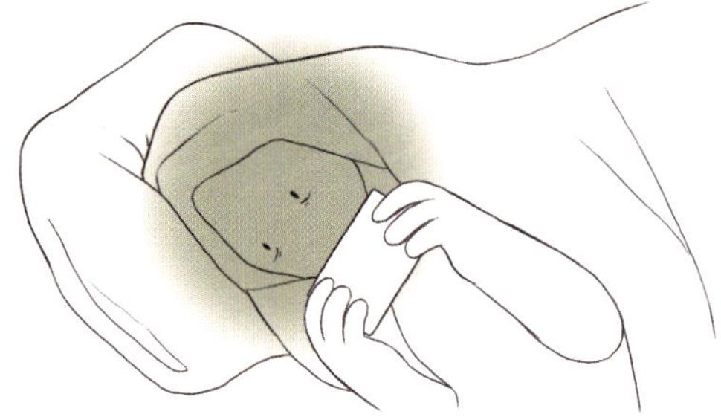

When we avoid activities or try to distract ourselves, we may make our depression worse.

Here are some examples of healthy coping strategies. Circle the ones you enjoy. If you think of other ideas, write them in the blank boxes.

bicycling	walking	talking with a friend	meditating
gardening	stretching/yoga	doing art	doing sports
taking a bath	playing with a child/pet	spending time outdoors	eating/drinking healthily
writing in a journal	playing an instrument		

Now, list two healthy coping strategies from the table above (or others) that you *have done* or would *like to do*.

Healthy coping strategy 1: ________________________________

____

____

Healthy coping strategy 2: ________________________________

____

____

There are ways to change our coping strategies, but we're usually most successful when we take *small steps*.

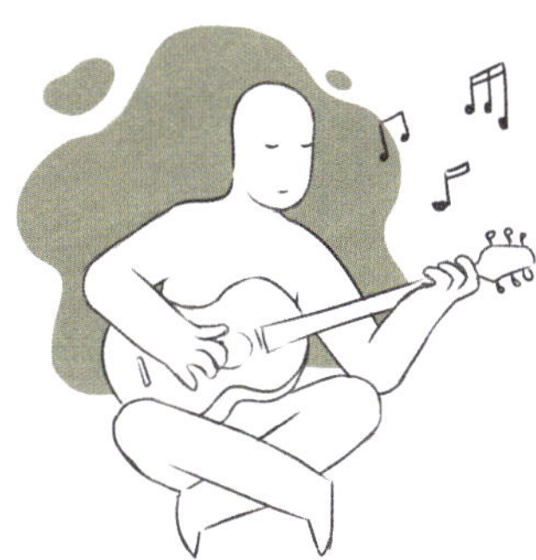

For example, maybe you eat more junk food when you're depressed, and you want to cut back. You could keep fewer chips and cookies at home, limit the amount you eat, or replace the sweets with more water, nuts, or sugarless gum. Or maybe you want to exercise more but often set yourself up for big changes only to have trouble maintaining them. Setting *reasonable goals* and building on them step by step will lead to better results.

If you wish to be more physically active, begin by walking twenty minutes a day, two days a week. Then gradually increase your walking time.

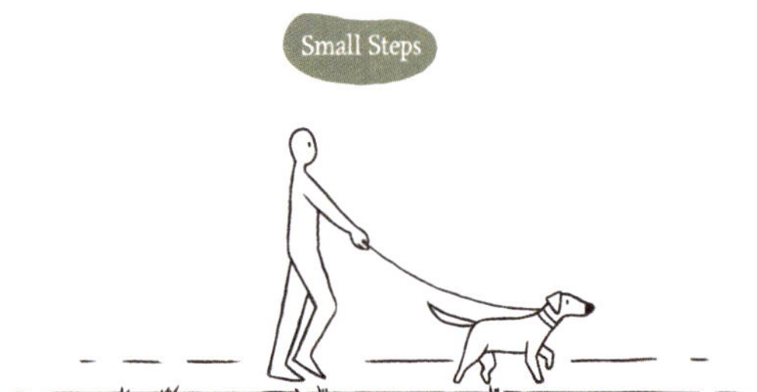

Any type of regular exercise has been shown time and again to have a positive effect on mood. When our mood brightens, we have more energy to do things that make us feel good.

What small steps will you take to start doing the two healthy coping strategies you just identified? List them here.

Small step 1: ______________________________

____

Small step 2: ______________________________

____

Set small, reasonable goals and congratulate yourself each time you meet one. Over time, you will really impact your depression.

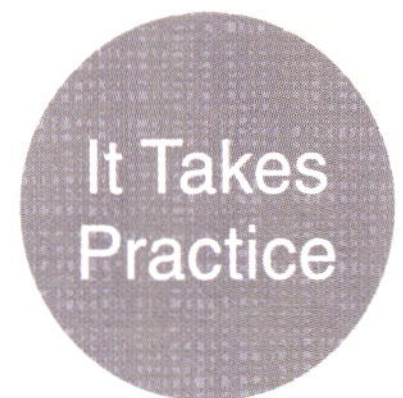

On your calendar, schedule the days you will be doing your new healthy coping strategy—like it's an appointment. Then be sure to keep that appointment with yourself. You're worth it!

EXERCISE 16

Healthy Sleep for Depression

When we don't sleep well or have disrupted sleep, we're more likely to become depressed. And when we're depressed, we often don't sleep well. It's a vicious cycle.

Here are some common issues that affect our sleep. Check the ones that apply to you.

- ☐ I have trouble falling asleep.
- ☐ I wake up in the night and can't fall back asleep.
- ☐ I look at my clock throughout the night.
- ☐ I watch TV, use my phone, or take my laptop to bed.
- ☐ I take naps during the day or spend a lot of time in bed.
- ☐ I'm groggy when I wake up and hit "snooze" many times.
- ☐ My partner keeps me awake (snoring, leaving lights on, etc.).
- ☐ I often have a drink before I go to bed.
- ☐ I smoke products with nicotine in the evening.
- ☐ I drink coffee or caffeinated sodas in the evening.

Answer the following questions.

How many days a week do you wake up feeling refreshed? Circle one.

0 1 2 3 4 5 6 7

What do you notice about your emotions when you don't get enough sleep?

In the table below, list what you think you can and can't control about your sleep habits. An example is provided for you.

When it comes to how well I sleep . . .	
I can control	**I can't control**
what time I go to bed	*the neighbors' noise*

Here are a few "sleep hygiene" practices we can use to get a better night's sleep:

- Follow a consistent routine—go to bed and wake up the same time each day.
- Avoid alcohol, caffeine, and nicotine in the evenings—they disrupt sleep.
- "Wind down" before you go to bed—listen to soothing music, dim the lights, or take a warm bath.
- Avoid using electronic devices—the computer, TV, and phone—within two hours of bedtime.
- Turn your clock to the wall—lying awake worrying about sleep you're not getting isn't helpful.
- Reduce noise as much as you can—earplugs can be helpful.
- Sleep in a cool room with air movement. A fan can help circulate air and keep you cool.
- Spend time in direct sunlight each day—aim for at least thirty minutes of exposure so your body understands the difference between day and night.
- Don't exercise right before bed. Be active during the day and calm in the evening.

Many of us struggle with insomnia—waking up for hours in the middle of the night or having trouble falling asleep. With depression, it can be hard to quiet our thoughts. We also might worry about the problems a poor night's sleep will cause us. This doesn't help! Here are some tips if we're struggling to fall and stay asleep.

- If you really can't sleep, get out of bed. It's best to use your bed only for sleep and get up and go to another room to read, stretch, or do a calming practice.
- Breathing exercises can be helpful. Try counting to four as you inhale and eight as you exhale.
- Guided meditation is useful. Several meditations are available online.
- Acknowledge your thoughts. Instead of trying to ignore them, you can say to yourself, "Now I'm thinking about ____________" or "I'm having a thought about ____________." Simply recognizing thoughts instead of trying to control them may help us relax and rest.

In this table, list your top problems with sleep. Then list steps you can take to address them.

Sleep Problem	Steps I Can Take

Practicing sleep hygiene skills can help us manage depression. When we're rested, we're less likely to dwell on negative thoughts and better able to accept events as they come.

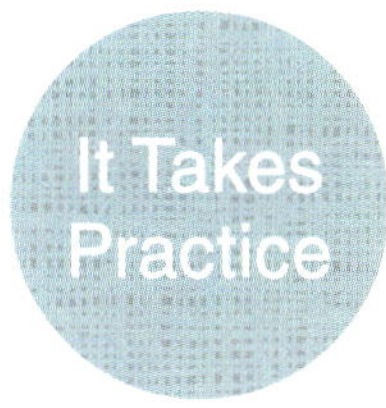

Choose one new sleep hygiene practice to try for a week. When it has become part of your routine, add another.

Managing Depression Effectively

SECTION 4

Whether we practice mindfulness, reach out to others, or look for a therapist to help us manage our depression, there are many strategies that can help us.

EXERCISE 17

Positive Affirmations

When we dwell on negative thoughts, we give them a lot of power. Repeating them over and over to ourselves makes them more automatic. But the opposite is true too! Repeating positive, more accurate thoughts in our heads can make them automatic.

Such phrases are called "affirmations" because they build a positive frame of mind. Here are some examples of affirmations.

"I am all right."

"I am on the right path for me."

"I am a good person, even if I make mistakes."

"I am cared about."

"I am starting to make better decisions."

"I have done well, and I will continue to do well."

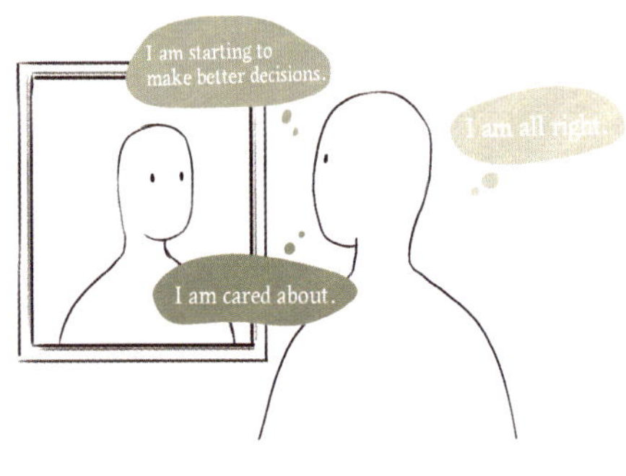

We can write our own personal affirmations. To start, complete the phrase "I am . . ." Keep the phrase short, positive, and realistic.

I am ____

____

I am ____

____

I am ____

____

Now write some positive affirmations about your life by completing the phrase "My life is . . ."

My life is ______________________________

____

____

My life is ______________________________

____

____

My life is ______________________________

____

____

If you have trouble coming up with positive affirmations, ask a person you trust to help you. By focusing on these positive affirmations, we squeeze out our negative, unhelpful thoughts. How you use affirmations is up to you, but they can be a powerful strategy against depression.

"If your compassion does not include yourself, it is incomplete."

—Jack Kornfield

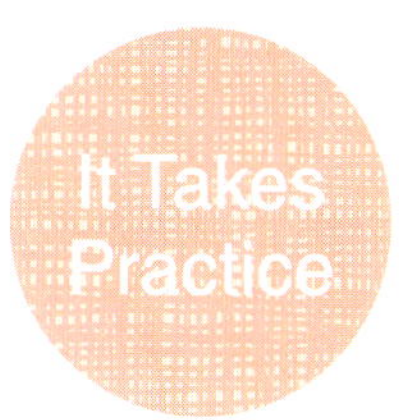

Affirmations are most effective when we say them to ourselves regularly. Write them down. Put them on sticky notes and place them on your bathroom mirror, on your refrigerator, or in your car. You could also write them in a journal and review them daily.

EXERCISE 18

Staying Present

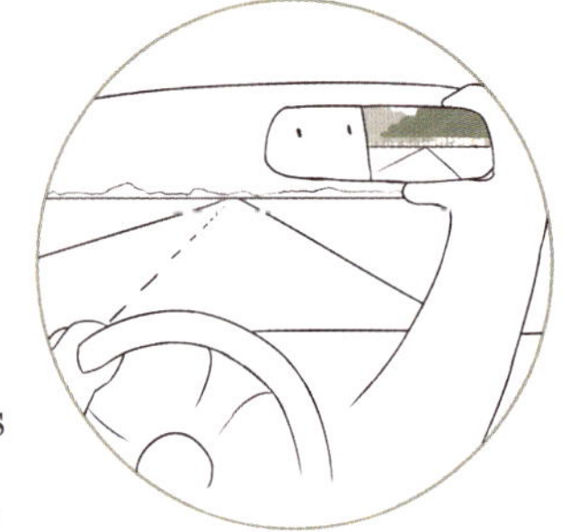

It's common, when we're depressed, to feel like we're caught in the past. As if we are staring in a rearview mirror, we dwell on what has happened and what we've done instead of focusing on the possibilities of the present moment.

Finding ways to stay present can help us appreciate what is happening right now, which strengthens our ability to push back against depression.

The following three techniques can help:

Grounding | Focused breathing | Mindfulness

Grounding focuses our attention on our senses in the moment. This helps us get out of the negative thoughts we repeat to ourselves. When we're grounding ourselves, we focus on what we can touch, hear, see, and smell. Sit in a comfortable position and ask yourself these questions:

Touch: What surfaces can your body feel right now? Focus on your feet touching the floor, your arms touching your side, your seat on the chair or bed. Where do you sense touch?

Sound: What do you hear around you? Tune in to the sounds in the room. Can you hear outside the room as well? What sounds can you hear?

Sight: Is it bright or dark? What do you see around you? What colors or objects do you see? Can you identify and count the number of red, green, white, or yellow items within your view?

Smell: What scents are you aware of? Can you smell anything in particular?

What emotions are you feeling after doing this grounding exercise?

How do these emotions compare to how you were feeling beforehand?

Focused breathing helps to clear the mind and relax the body. There are many breathing techniques, but one simple method is to count to ten:

1. Breathing through your nose, draw a deep breath all the way into your belly. Allow the belly to fill gently.
2. Count "one."
3. Exhale slowly through your mouth.
4. Pause and count "two."
5. Inhale again through the nose and down into the belly on the "odd" breath count.
6. Exhale through the mouth on the "even" breath count.
7. Repeat until you reach a count of ten.
8. Repeat this process as many times as you need to until you're feeling calmer and more focused.

Mindfulness helps us practice being "present." It's a way of observing what we're doing right now, without distractions or judgment. It's meant to help us accept where we are, without thinking about what has happened or what will happen next.

You can practice mindfulness while doing everyday activities. Here are some examples:

- **When you're walking, focus just on your walking.** How do your shoes feel? What do you see? How does the air feel? What do you smell?
- **When you're driving your car, focus just on your driving.** What does the seat feel like? How fast are you going? What are the road conditions?
- **When you're eating a meal, focus just on your eating.** How does the food taste? How does it feel to chew the food? What aromas do you smell?

You may find that other thoughts creep in as you're practicing mindfulness. Don't struggle with them. Like clouds in the sky, let them float in and out as you gently bring your focus back to the here and now.

You can practice mindfulness with any simple activity that you enjoy, such as cooking, walking, exercising, or petting your dog or cat.

Practicing these three techniques—grounding, focused breathing, and mindfulness—can help us manage our depression. And the great thing is, we can use these techniques anytime, anywhere! If we're paying attention to the here and now, we're not acting on our negative thoughts or worries.

"Mindfulness is a way of befriending ourselves and our experience."

—Jon Kabat-Zinn

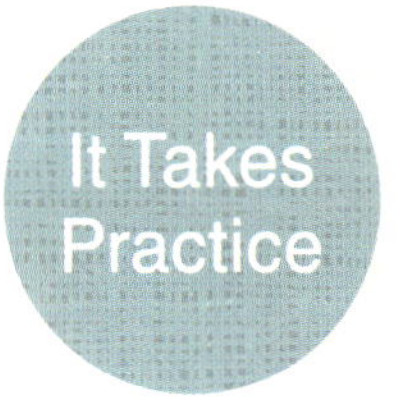

Commit to practicing one of these techniques every day. Eventually it will become automatic to use them when needed.

EXERCISE 19

Reaching Out

We tend to isolate when we're depressed. But no one is an island. We can—and should—reach out to others for emotional support.

Think about all the people you know in each area of your life. Who would be open to talking with you? Whom would you like to talk with?

Someone at *home:* ______________________

Someone at *work* or *school:* ______________________

Someone I think of as a *counselor:* ______________________

Someone I think of as a *mentor:* ______________________

Someone I think of as a *friend:* ______________________

Consider whether you'd like to get their advice or hear their perspective. Maybe you'd just like to talk, nothing too heavy.

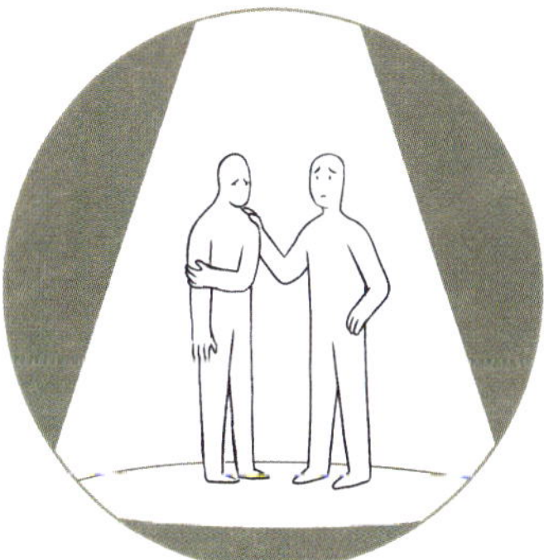

It can be hard to reach out when you're depressed, but remind yourself that *you matter.* And people are often flattered when others contact them, whether it's for advice or to simply say hello.

To make this easier, try

- taking a deep breath
- thinking of what this person means to you
- thinking of good conversations the two of you have had before
- taking one small step to reach out to them

Open yourself up to listening as well as talking. Keep breathing. And keep in mind that while texting, emailing, and using social media are great ways to reach out, talking on the phone, using video chat, and meeting face-to-face allow for a deeper personal connection.

Building support doesn't just have to be one-on-one. You can reach out to groups you've been a part of or might be interested in. You can return to activities you've enjoyed.

What groups or activities have you enjoyed in the past?

What new groups or activities sound interesting to you?

What is one goal you could set that would help you reach out more to others for support?

If we struggle with depression, we can often feel like not reaching out, but so often we feel better when we do. Reaching out is key to fighting depression and building a healthy life.

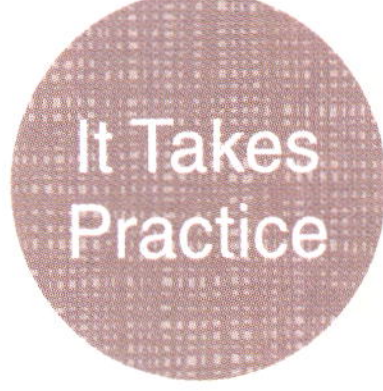

Each week, identify one person to reach out to and contact them.

EXERCISE 20

Communicating Well

Sometimes our depression can be negatively affected by conflicts with people. Many of these conflicts develop when we don't know how to

- listen well
- ask for what we want
- express appreciation

The good news is these skills can be developed. By learning to communicate more effectively, we can take further control of our depression.

Listen Fully

Skilled listeners do more than simply hear people's words. They pick up on nonverbal things like the person's gestures, posture, and tone of voice. These things often say more than words alone. This is listening fully.

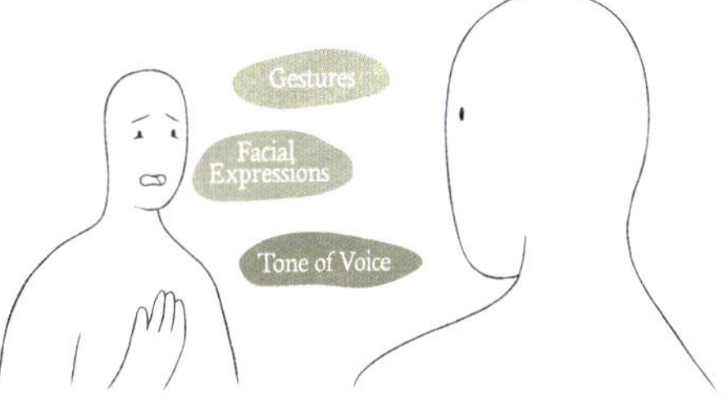

When we listen fully, we create a safe space for people to talk. They can then let down their defenses, open up, and share what they're truly thinking and feeling. In turn, they'll be more willing to listen fully when it's your turn to talk.

Specific things you can do to listen fully include the following:

1. Maintain eye contact with the person who's talking.
2. Adjust your posture to show you're open to listening—for example, uncross your arms and legs and sit closer to the speaker.
3. Allow people to express emotions—to cry, shout, or do anything else, as long as it doesn't affect your personal safety.
4. Keep silent while the other person is speaking. Don't interrupt. Allow people to keep talking until they're done. Then follow up by asking, "Is there anything else you'd like to say?"
5. Resist the urge to respond immediately with your own opinions or suggestions.

Ask for What You Want

This means stating your thoughts and feelings without blaming or shaming anyone. It also means being honest and saying what you need.

Use these three phrases in order:

I see . . .

I feel . . .

I want . . .

I see your stuff all over the table.
I feel overwhelmed by clutter.
I want us to keep the house clean.

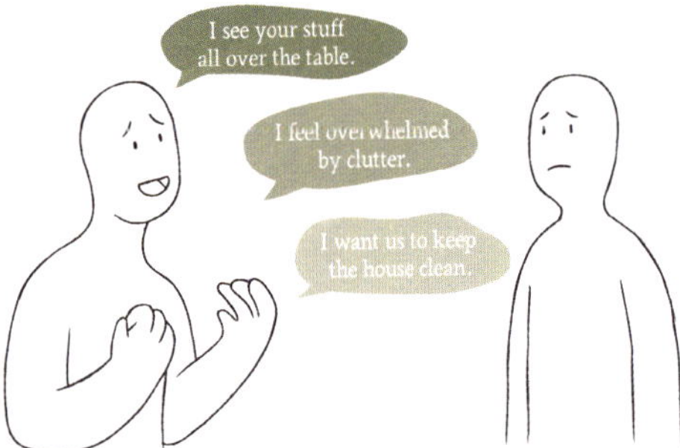

The first phrase—**I see**—means you state the facts about a situation. By speaking to the facts, you prevent arguments (you avoid hearing "That's just *your* opinion").

The second phrase—**I feel**—helps you link your feelings to the facts. The goal is to simply say what's going on inside you.

With the third phrase—**I want**—you ask for one specific change. Ask for changes in *behavior* rather than attitudes or emotions. People can change what they do more easily than they can change what they think or feel.

Your request will be more powerful if you state the benefits of making this change, emphasize your willingness to participate, and express appreciation.

• • •

Let's try out this formula. Suppose you live with someone who often leaves dirty dishes in the kitchen sink. Here is how you might address it:

> *Can I talk to you for a second about the dishes?* ***I see*** *dirty dishes in the sink when I go to the kitchen.* ***I feel*** *uncomfortable with this.* ***I want*** *us to wash the dishes after each meal. This would make our kitchen a lot easier to work in. I'm willing to do my share, and I'd really appreciate it if you could too.*

Think about a conversation you'd like to have with someone about an issue. Write it out in the space on the next page. Practice saying it out loud to someone before you approach the person it's meant for.

My Conversation . . .

Hi, can I talk to you for a second about ______________________________

____

____?

I see ____

____

____.

I feel ____

____

____.

I'd like/I want ____

____

____

____.

Express Appreciation

When someone does something you appreciate—no matter how small the deed—say *thanks.* Showing gratitude like this can actually increase our level of happiness.

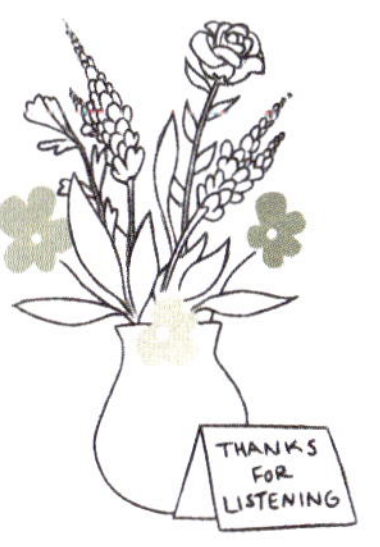

Instead of focusing on the things people do wrong, make a special effort to notice when they do things right.

Think about kind things people have recently done for you. Write one or two statements below that express your gratitude.

____

____

____

EXERCISE 21

What about Therapy?

It can be helpful to talk with someone trained to assist us with depression if we aren't doing so already. Psychotherapy can be effective for many reasons. There's a saying: "If you can mention it, then you can manage it." Simply telling someone what you've been thinking and feeling can help you feel better.

A therapist can also help you discover patterns in your thoughts and behaviors that are hard to see on your own. Once you see these patterns, you can choose to change them in a supportive setting.

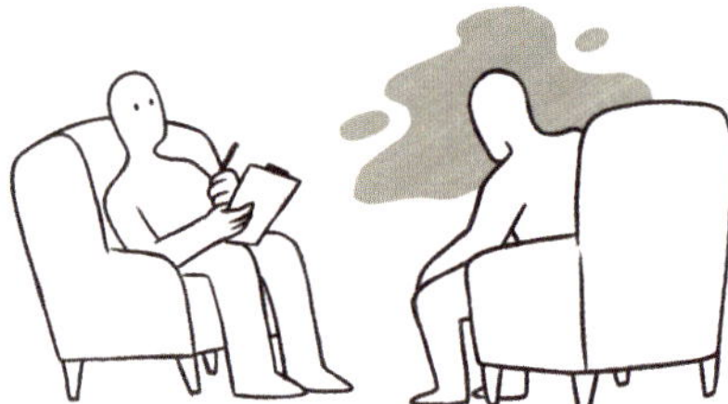

Types of Psychotherapists

Psychiatrists, psychologists, social workers, and other trained counselors can offer therapy. Only licensed physicians, such as a primary care provider or a psychiatrist, can prescribe medication.

Tips to Keep in Mind

Financial	Personal
Before you begin looking for a therapist, see if your insurance will pay for it. Your coverage may also limit whom you can see.	Ask for referrals—your physician could recommend a therapist. Trusted friends or family members may also have recommendations.
If you don't have insurance, check out your county or community mental health departments. They may know of low-cost or no-cost options.	Find a therapist by doing an internet search using terms like "mental health," "psychotherapy," "counseling," "social services," or "crisis intervention services."
If you live by a college or university, its medical school or psychology department may offer mental health services on a sliding-fee scale.	Consider what you're looking for in a therapist. Some people feel more comfortable with male counselors; some with female. You may want to see a therapist who specializes in a specific area, such as gender identity, relationships, trauma, or life transitions.

Some people need to take medication for depression to feel better. A psychiatrist can prescribe antidepressants; your primary doctor may be able to as well. Talk with your therapist about whether medications may help. When taking medications, be sure to follow instructions and check in regularly with the physician prescribing them.

List any financial concerns you have regarding therapy.

Where might you look for a therapist?

What qualities in a therapist are most important to you? Consider gender, location, and specialty. List them below.

"If you can mention it, then you can manage it."

—Fred Rogers

If you're in crisis, go to a local emergency room. Professionals there can refer you to further help.

Questions to Ask

It's important that you can relate to and feel comfortable with the therapist. Ask questions before you commit to several sessions. If, after a few visits, you don't feel like you're making a connection, switch to a different provider. The goal is to find someone who's a good fit for *you*. Therapists will respect your right to be a smart consumer.

Here are some questions to ask:

1. How long have you been in practice?
2. What approach will you use to treat problems related to depression?
3. How long do your clients typically stay in therapy?
4. How many times per week or month will I see you?
5. Can you prescribe medications or refer me to someone who can?
6. If you take time off or if I have an emergency when you're not working, how can I get help?

List other questions you might have below.

To get the most from therapy, respond openly and honestly to your therapist's questions. Be willing to consider new ideas. Keep your appointments, even when you don't feel like going. And remember to do any assigned "homework" between sessions.

It takes time to feel better—therapy doesn't offer an "instant cure." Talk to your therapist about identifying the signs of progress and set realistic goals together.

EXERCISE 22

Goals and Strategies for Managing Depression

There is hope. We don't overcome depression overnight, but there are many things we can do to feel better. Here are some ideas we've discussed in this workbook:

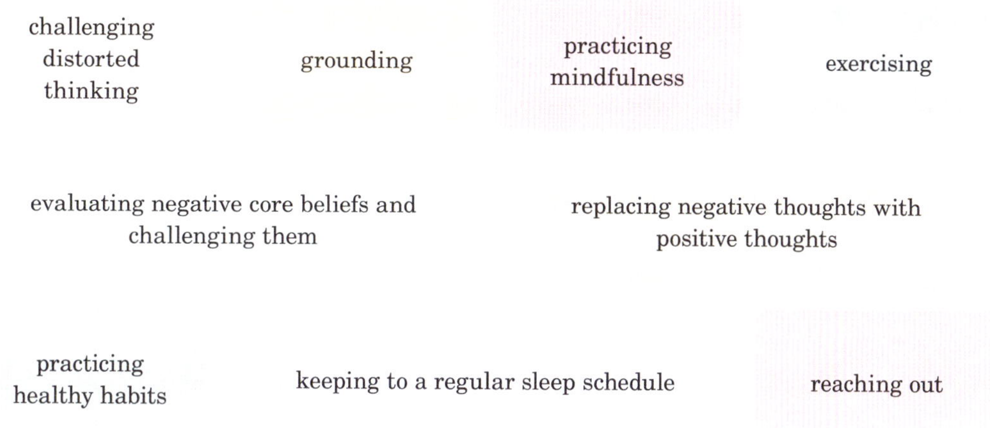

Depression is an individual experience—you may find some strategies work better than others. Regardless of what works best for you, it's important to set goals.

Set some personal goals for managing your depression by completing the table below. An example is done for you.

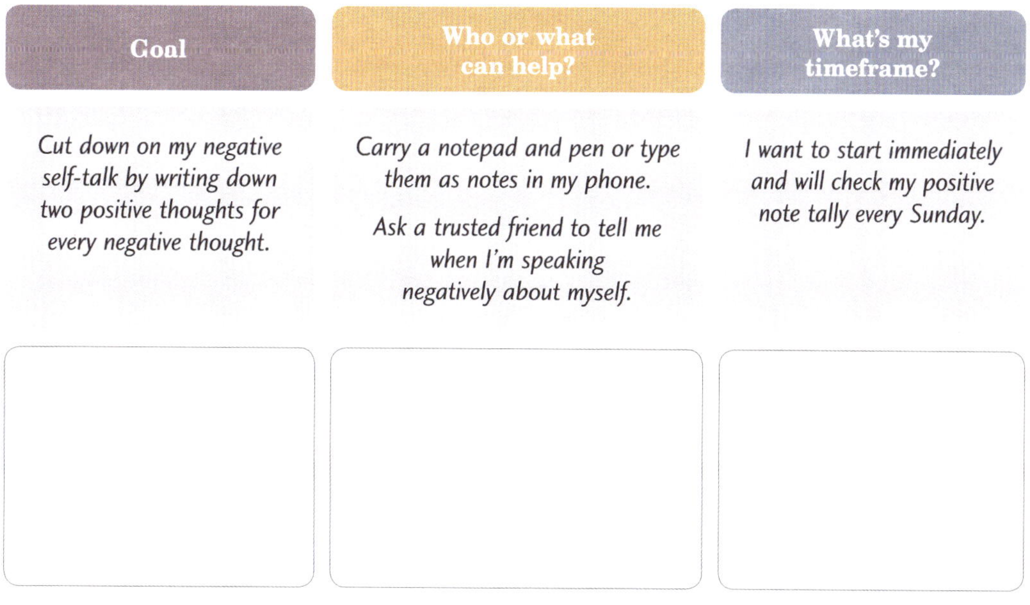

Goal	Who or what can help?	What's my timeframe?
Cut down on my negative self-talk by writing down two positive thoughts for every negative thought.	*Carry a notepad and pen or type them as notes in my phone.* *Ask a trusted friend to tell me when I'm speaking negatively about myself.*	*I want to start immediately and will check my positive note tally every Sunday.*

table continued on next page

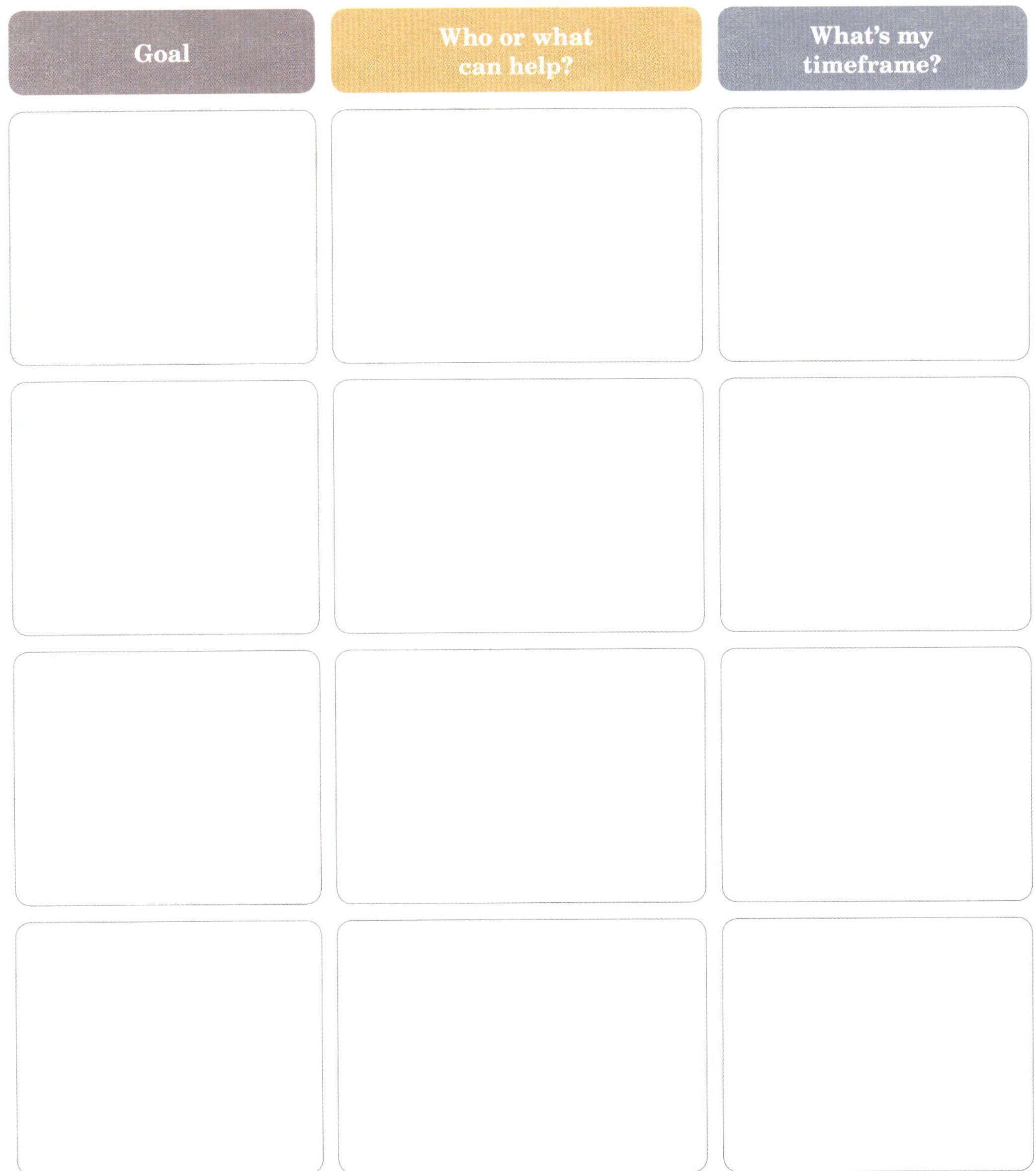

Goal	Who or what can help?	What's my timeframe?

The best way to make changes is to start slowly and build over time. Each of these strategies can help us build our confidence, reduce our depression, and live more fully.

"Hold on to this hope: You can get better from depression."

—HealthyPlace.com

My Notes

My Notes

About this workbook

Many exercises in this workbook are based on therapeutic approaches from cognitive-behavioral therapy (CBT), acceptance and commitment therapy (ACT), and dialectical behavior therapy (DBT).

CBT is based on the theory that human thoughts and feelings influence human behavior. It aims to help individuals change their thought patterns in order to change their responses to circumstances. CBT was pioneered in the 1960s by Aaron Beck and remains widely practiced. Refer to *Cognitive Therapy and the Emotional Disorders* by Aaron T. Beck (New York: Penguin Books, 1979).

ACT and DBT were developed in the 1980s by Steven Hayes and Marsha Linehan, respectively. An empirically validated intervention, ACT combines acceptance and mindfulness strategies with commitment and behavior change approaches to increase an individual's psychological flexibility and ability to stay mentally present. More information can be found in *Learning ACT: An Acceptance and Commitment Therapy Skills-Training Manual for Therapists,* second edition, by Jason B. Luoma, Steven C. Hayes, and Robyn D. Walser (Oakland, CA: Context Press, 2017).

DBT emphasizes therapeutic skill-building in four key areas: mindfulness, distress tolerance, emotion regulation, and interpersonal effectiveness. See *DBT Skills Training Manual,* second edition, 1993, and also (available separately) *DBT Skills Training Handouts and Worksheets,* second edition, 2015, both by Marsha M. Linehan (New York: Guilford Press).

Notes

1. In Exercise 11: Distorted Thinking, pages 27–28, the thinking distortions originally come from David Burns, MD, adapted from *Feeling Good: The New Mood Therapy* (New York: William Morrow & Company, 1980; Signet, 1981)

2. In Exercise 19: Reaching Out, page 49, "But no one is an island" paraphrases "But no man is an island," which comes from "Meditation XVII," *Devotions Upon Emergent Occasions,* by John Donne, written in 1623.

3. In Exercise 21: What about Therapy?, page 55, the quote "If you can mention it, then you can manage it" is adapted from Fred Rogers, interview by John Callaway, *Chicago Tonight,* 1985, video posted on PBS website, December 26, 2019, https://www.pbs.org/video/archives-fred-rogers-interview-john-callaway-8texm7.

About Hazelden Publishing

As part of the Hazelden Betty Ford Foundation, Hazelden Publishing offers both cutting-edge educational resources and inspirational books. Our print and digital works help guide individuals in treatment and recovery, and their loved ones. Professionals who work to prevent and treat addiction also turn to Hazelden Publishing for evidence-based curricula, digital content solutions, and videos for use in schools, treatment programs, correctional programs, and electronic health records systems. We also offer training for implementation of our curricula.

Through published and digital works, Hazelden Publishing extends the reach of healing and hope to individuals, families, and communities affected by addiction and related issues.

For more information about Hazelden publications, please call **800-328-9000** or visit us online at **hazelden.org/bookstore**.

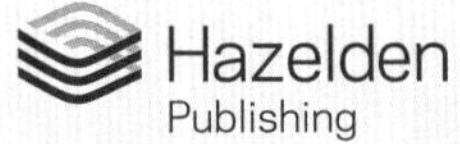

Center City, Minnesota 55012
hazelden.org/bookstore

ISBN: 978-1-61649-937-2

Editor's notes:

This publication is not intended as a substitute for the advice of health care professionals. Several activities in this workbook are based on therapeutic approaches from cognitive-behavioral therapy, acceptance and commitment therapy, and dialectical behavior therapy.

Readers should be aware that websites listed in this work may have changed or disappeared between when this work was written and when it is read.

Hazelden Publishing offers a variety of information on addiction and related areas. The views and interpretations expressed herein are those of the author and are neither endorsed nor approved by Alcoholics Anonymous (AA) or any Twelve Step organization.

Cover designer: *Theresa Jaeger Gedig*
Interior designer, typesetter: *Terri Kinne*
Author: *Marshall Robinson, PhD*
Developmental editors: *Abigail Karels, Sue Thomas*
Content project managers: *Anita Dincesen, Abigail Karels*
Editorial project managers: *April Ebb, Jean Cook*

Illustrators: *Anna Faught, Shelby Pearson, Chris Handrick*

Subject-matter experts:
Deborah L. Mosby, MS, LADC, MAC
Princess Drake, MS, PsyD